Global Oral and Maxillofacial Surgery

Editors

SHAHID R. AZIZ
JOSE M. MARCHENA
STEVEN M. ROSER

ORAL AND MAXILLOFACIAL SURGERY CLINICS OF NORTH AMERICA

www.oralmaxsurgery.theclinics.com

Consulting Editor
RUI P. FERNANDES

August 2020 • Volume 32 • Number 3

ELSEVIER

1600 John F. Kennedy Boulevard • Suite 1800 • Philadelphia, Pennsylvania, 19103-2899

http://www.oralmaxsurgery.theclinics.com

ORAL AND MAXILLOFACIAL SURGERY CLINICS OF NORTH AMERICA Volume 32, Number 3
August 2020 ISSN 1042-3699, ISBN-13: 978-0-323-71080-0

Editor: John Vassallo; j.vassallo@elsevier.com
Developmental Editor: Laura Fisher

Oral and Maxillofacial Surgery Clinics of North America (ISSN 1042-3699) is published quarterly by Elsevier Inc., 360 Park Avenue South, New York, NY 10010-1710. Months of issue are February, May, August, and November. Business and Editorial Offices: 1600 John F. Kennedy Blvd., Suite 1800, Philadelphia, PA 19103-2899. Periodicals postage paid at New York, NY and additional mailing offices. Subscription prices are $401.00 per year for US individuals, $756.00 per year for US institutions, $100.00 per year for US students/residents, $474.00 per year for Canadian individuals, $906.00 per year for Canadian institutions, $100.00 per year for Canadian students/residents, $525.00 per year for international individuals, $906.00 per year for international institutions and $235.00 per year for international students/residents. To receive student/resident rate, orders must be accompanied by name or affiliated institution, date of term, and the *signature* of program/residency coordinator on institution letterhead. Orders will be billed at individual rate until proof of status is received. Foreign air speed delivery is included in all *Clinics* subscription prices. All prices are subject to change without notice. **POSTMASTER:** Send address changes to *Oral and Maxillofacial Surgery Clinics of North America* Elsevier Periodicals **Customer Service, 11830 Westline Industrial Drive, St. Louis, MO 63146. Tel: 1-800-654-2452 (U.S. and Canada); 314-447-8871 (outside U.S. and Canada). Fax: 314-447-8029. E-mail: journalscustomerservice-usa@elsevier.com (for print support); journalsonlinesupport-usa@elsevier.com (for online support).**

Reprints. For copies of 100 or more, of articles in this publication, please contact the Commercial Reprints Department, Elsevier Inc., 360 Park Avenue South, New York, NY 10010-1710. Tel.: 212-633-3874; Fax: 212-633-3820; Email: reprints@elsevier.com.

Oral and Maxillofacial Surgery Clinics of North America is covered in *MEDLINE/PubMed* (*Index Medicus*), *Science Citation Index Expanded (SciSearch®)*, *Journal Citation Reports/Science Edition*, and *Current Contents®/Clinical Medicine*.

Contributors

CONSULTING EDITOR

RUI P. FERNANDES, MD, DMD, FACS, FRCS(Ed)
Clinical Professor and Chief, Division of Head and Neck Surgery, Program Director, Head and Neck Oncologic Surgery and Microvascular Reconstruction Fellowship, Departments of Oral and Maxillofacial Surgery, Neurosurgery, and Orthopaedic Surgery and Rehabilitation, University of Florida Health Science Center, University of Florida College of Medicine, Jacksonville, Florida, USA

EDITORS

SHAHID R. AZIZ, DMD MD, FACS, FRCS(Ed)
Assistant Dean of Global Health, Professor, Department of Oral and Maxillofacial Surgery, Rutgers School of Dental Medicine, Associate Professor, Division of Plastic and Reconstructive Surgery, Department of Surgery, Rutgers New Jersey Medical School, Newark, New Jersey, USA; Visiting Professor, Update Dental College, Dhaka, Bangladesh; Founder and President, Smile Bangladesh, Mountainside, New Jersey, USA

JOSE M. MARCHENA, DMD, MD, FACS
Associate Professor, Department of Oral and Maxillofacial Surgery, The University of Texas Health Science Center at Houston, School of Dentistry, Chief of Oral and Maxillofacial Surgery, Ben Taub Hospital, Houston, Texas, USA; Visiting Professor, Update Dental College, Dhaka, Bangladesh; Vice President, Smile Bangladesh, Mountainside, New Jersey, USA

STEVEN M. ROSER, DMD, MD, FACS, FRCS(Ed)
DeLos Hill Chair and Professor of Surgery, Chief, Division of Oral and Maxillofacial Surgery, Chair, Emory Perioperative Global Health Group, Department of Surgery, Emory University School of Medicine, Atlanta, Georgia, USA; Team Leader, Healing the Children, Northeast, Chair, Committee on Global Surgery, Permanent Council Member, G4 Alliance, International Association of Oral and Maxillofacial Surgery Foundation

AUTHORS

SALIM AFSHAR, MD, DMD
Program in Global Surgery and Social Change, Harvard Medical School, Department of Plastic and Oral Surgery, Boston Children's Hospital, Harvard School of Dental Medicine, Boston, Massachusetts, USA

SHAHID R. AZIZ, DMD MD, FACS, FRCS(Ed)
Assistant Dean of Global Health, Professor, Department of Oral and Maxillofacial Surgery, Rutgers School of Dental Medicine, Associate Professor, Division of Plastic and Reconstructive

Surgery, Department of Surgery, Rutgers New Jersey Medical School, Newark, New Jersey, USA; Visiting Professor, Update Dental College, Dhaka, Bangladesh; Founder and President, Smile Bangladesh, Mountainside, New Jersey, USA

JAMES E. BERTZ, DDS, MD, FACS
Professor Emeritus, Department of Oral and Maxillofacial Surgery, The University of Texas Health Science Center at Houston, Houston, Texas, USA

MATTHEW J. DAVIS, BS
Division of Plastic Surgery, Department of Surgery, Texas Children's Hospital, Michael E. DeBakey Department of Surgery, Baylor College of Medicine, Houston, Texas, USA

RACHEL W. DAVIS, MD
Founder, Integrated Global Surgery Track, Michael E. DeBakey Department of Surgery, Baylor College of Medicine, Houston, Texas, USA

NAGI DEMIAN, DDS, MD, FACS
Professor, Department of Oral and Maxillofacial Surgery, The University of Texas Health Science Center at Houston, School of Dentistry, Houston, Texas, USA

PRIYA DESAI, MPH
Smile Train, New York, New York, USA

WILLIAM FOEGE, MD, MPH
Professor Emeritus, Rollins School of Public Health, Emory University, Director Emeritus, Centers for Disease Control, Health Policy Fellow, The Carter Center, Atlanta, Georgia

GHALI E. GHALI, DDS, MD, FACS, FRCSEd
Professor and Chairman, Department of Oral and Maxillofacial Surgery, LSU Health Sciences Center, Chancellor, Louisiana State University Health System, Shreveport, Louisiana, USA

EVONNE GREENIDGE, MD
Secretary, Smile Bangladesh, Mountainside, New Jersey, USA; Pediatric Anesthesiologist, Private Practice, Washington, DC, USA

MARY M. GULLATTE, PhD, RN, ANP-BC, AOCN, FAAN
Corporate Director, Nursing Research and Evidence Based Practice, Emory Healthcare, Inc, Atlanta, Georgia, USA

HUSSEIN K. HAJI, BSc Pharm, RPH, DDS
Toronto, Ontario, Canada

DAVID HOFFMAN, DDS, FACS
Department of Oral and Maxillofacial Surgery, Staten Island Oral Surgery, Staten Island, New York, USA

LARRY H. HOLLIER JR, MD
Division of Plastic Surgery, Department of Surgery, Texas Children's Hospital, Michael E. DeBakey Department of Surgery, Baylor College of Medicine, Houston, Texas, USA

ORESTE IOCCA, DDS, MD
Research Fellow, Department of Otolaryngology–Head and Neck Surgery, Humanitas Clinical and Research Center, IRCCS, Milano, Italy

MICHAEL KRIEVES, MD
Pediatric Anesthesiologist, Private Practice, Grand Junction, Colorado, USA; Team Anesthesia Leader, Smile Bangladesh, Mountainside, New Jersey, USA

KENNETH KUFTA, DMD, MD
Resident in Oral and Maxillofacial Surgery, School of Dental Medicine, University of Pennsylvania, Perelman Center for Advanced Medicine, Philadelphia, Pennsylvania, USA

JESSICA S. LEE, DDS, MD, MA
Fellow, Pediatric Cleft and Craniofacial Surgery, Cleft and Craniofacial Center, Charleston Area Medical Center Women and Children's Hospital, Charleston, West Virginia, USA

VICTORIA A. MAÑÓN, DDS
Resident, Department of Oral and Maxillofacial Surgery, The University of Texas Health Science Center at Houston, School of Dentistry, Houston, Texas, USA

JOSE M. MARCHENA, DMD, MD, FACS
Associate Professor, Department of Oral and Maxillofacial Surgery, The University of Texas Health Science Center at Houston, School of

Dentistry, Chief of Oral and Maxillofacial Surgery, Ben Taub Hospital, Houston, Texas, USA; Visiting Professor, Update Dental College, Dhaka, Bangladesh; Vice President, Smile Bangladesh, Mountainside, New Jersey, USA

JOHN G. MEARA, MD, DMD, MBA
Program in Global Surgery and Social Change, Harvard Medical School, Department of Plastic and Oral Surgery, Boston Children's Hospital, Boston, Massachusetts, USA

MOTIUR RAHMAN MOLLA, BDS, PhD, FCPS, Dip – OMS, FICS, FICD
Head, Department of Oral and Maxillofacial Surgery, Anwer Khan Modern Medical College and Hospital, Dhanmondi, Dhaka, Bangladesh

NAFISA MARIUM MOLLA, BDS, DDS
Toronto, Ontario, Canada

VENNILA PADMANABAN, MD
Department of Surgery, Rutgers New Jersey Medical School, Newark, New Jersey, USA

ROLVIX H. PATTERSON, MD, MPH
Program in Global Surgery and Social Change, Harvard Medical School, Tufts University School of Medicine, Boston, Massachusetts, USA

KATE PETTORINI, MSN, RN, CNOR
Unit Nurse Educator, Operating Room, Emory University Hospital a Magnet™ Designated Facility, Atlanta, Georgia, USA

QUAZI BILLUR RAHMAN, MD, PGD, PhD
Professor and Chair, Department of Oral and Maxillofacial Surgery, Bangabandhu Sheikh Mujib Medical University, Dhaka, Bangladesh

CHÉ L. REDDY, MBChB, MPH
Program in Global Surgery and Social Change, Harvard Medical School, Department of Plastic and Oral Surgery, Boston Children's Hospital, Boston, Massachusetts, USA

STEVEN M. ROSER, DMD, MD, FACS, FRCS(Ed)
DeLos Hill Chair and Professor of Surgery, Chief, Division of Oral and Maxillofacial Surgery, Chair, Emory Perioperative Global Health Group, Department of Surgery, Emory University School of Medicine, Atlanta, Georgia, USA; Team Leader, Healing the Children, Northeast, Chair, Committee on Global Surgery, Permanent Council Member, G4 Alliance, International Association of Oral and Maxillofacial Surgery Foundation

CHRISTIAN SANDROCK, MD, MPH, FCCP
Professor of Medicine, Vice Chair, Quality and Safety, Clinical Chief, Division of Pulmonary and Critical Care Medicine, Division of Infectious Diseases, Department of Internal Medicine, UC Davis School of Medicine, Sacramento, California, USA

RABIE M. SHANTI, DMD, MD
Assistant Professor of Oral and Maxillofacial Surgery and Pharmacology, School of Dental Medicine, University of Pennsylvania, Perelman Center for Advanced Medicine, Philadelphia, Pennsylvania, USA

YOUMNA A. SHERIF, MD
Global Surgery Fellow, Michael E. DeBakey Department of Surgery, Baylor College of Medicine, Houston, Texas, USA

ZIAD C. SIFRI, MD, FACS
Department of Surgery, Rutgers New Jersey Medical School, Newark, New Jersey, USA

RENE SOLORZANO, CAT
Anesthesia Technician, Smile Bangladesh, Mountainside, New Jersey, USA; Certified Anesthesia Technician, Department of Anesthesiology, Columbia University Irving Medical Center, New York, New York, USA

ANGELA S. VOLK, MD
Division of Plastic Surgery, Department of Surgery, Texas Children's Hospital, Michael E. DeBakey Department of Surgery, Baylor College of Medicine, Houston, Texas, USA

ISAAC WASSERMAN, MD, MPH
Program in Global Surgery and Social Change, Harvard Medical School, Boston, Massachusetts, USA; Icahn School of Medicine at Mount Sinai, New York, New York, USA

THOMAS P. WILLIAMS, DDS, MD, FACS
Dubuque, Iowa, USA

Contents

Global health has evolved to focus on reducing health inequity and obtaining the highest attainable standard of health for all people. To do this, a range of actors now pursue interventions and policy with an eye toward global targets that place strong emphasis on improving health systems. Within global health, global surgery has sought to delineate the burden of surgical disease and propose policy to improve access to surgery. Oral and maxillofacial surgery has been underrepresented in global health but has a vital role in reducing the global health inequity attributable to the impact of oral and craniofacial conditions.

Five billion people worldwide do not have access to safe, affordable surgical and anesthesia care. The burden of inadequate access to safe and affordable surgical care falls heaviest on individuals living in low-income and middle-income countries (LMIC), where 9 out of 10 people do not have access to basic surgical care. Global oral and maxillofacial surgical care is included in the global burden of surgical disease, and increased awareness of the need for global oral and maxillofacial surgery (OMS), with the initiation, support, and funding of research on the need to develop a global OMS capacity-building strategy is imperative.

Head and neck cancer is increasing globally owing to rising rates of tobacco use and human papillomavirus infection. Today, cancer is the leading cause of death and disabilities in developed countries and the second leading cause of death in countries with developing economies. Understanding the global landscape of head and neck cancer will empower oral and maxillofacial surgeons to play a critical role among patients and societal education regarding the importance of addressing modifiable risk factors and continuing to play an important role in the diagnosis and management of head and neck cancer.

Since the introduction of oral and maxillofacial surgery in Southeast Asia, the field has expanded considerably in the region, with existing oral and maxillofacial surgeons performing a multitude of complex surgical procedures, ranging from orthognathic surgical procedures to oncological resection and reconstruction cases. Oral and maxillofacial surgery continues, however, to have considerable potential for growth in Southeast Asia. To accomplish this growth, assistance from the global oral surgery community has proved and continues to prove invaluable and essential.

Health disparities in the United States have been well documented over the past several decades and continue to affect the American population. As the world becomes more diverse, it is imperative that the health care professional workforce is trained to care for the diversifying patient population, striving to improve health disparities in the United States and worldwide. Improving the diversity within the health care professional workforce likely will aid in emphasizing the importance of cultural competency of health care professionals, with the development of programs aimed at cultural competency training and assessment.

International travel goes hand in hand with medical delivery to underserved communities. The global health care worker can be exposed to a wide range of infectious diseases during their global experiences. A pretravel risk assessment visit and all appropriate vaccinations and education must be performed. Universal practices of water safety, food safety, and insect avoidance will prevent most travel-related infections and complications. Region-specific vaccinations will further reduce illness risk. An understanding of common travel-related illness signs and symptoms is helpful. Emerging pathogens that can cause a pandemic should be understood to avoid health care worker infection and spread.

Anesthesia for oral and maxillofacial procedures during volunteer surgical missions requires careful planning of personnel, equipment, supplies, and coordination with the host medical institution. Cleft lip and palate repair are the most common oral and maxillofacial surgeries performed, and can be performed safely in low-resource environments when proper care and planning is taken.

There are marked disparities in supply and demand for specialty-trained health care providers in low-income and middle-income countries (LMIC). Nurses are at the forefront in volunteering to provide humanitarian health support in local, national, and international disasters. Responding to the call to provide expert medical and surgical education and care in LMIC aligns with the passion and purpose of nursing. This article shares a real-world experience of perioperative nurses in partnership with the surgical team to provide cleft lip/palate repair for children in LMIC. It is all in the smile left behind.

Formal Training of the Global Surgeon: Current Educational Paradigms and Critical Elements for Progression   447

Youmna A. Sherif and Rachel W. Davis

To prepare global surgeons, academic institutions have created training programs that provide opportunities to develop foundational clinical knowledge, pursue academic inquiry, build surgical infrastructure and capacity, and become advocates and collaborators in resource-limited settings. Academic institutions can create a short course in global surgery, global surgery rotation, global surgery fellowship, or integrated global surgery residency. Global surgery training programs must account for ethics of global surgery engagement, sources of funding, structures for professional advancement, and trainee-appropriate partnerships. Global surgery training must include the establishment of accreditation systems, development of integrated training programs, and institutional investment in global surgery education.

Answering the Call: How to Establish a Dentoalveolar Surgery Mission in Low- and Middle-Income Countries   457

Victoria A. Mañón, Nagi Demian, Shahid R. Aziz, and Jose M. Marchena

Addressing access to oral health care in many low- to middle-income countries is a complicated issue. Oral and maxillofacial surgeons may help engage with vulnerable populations through carefully planned dentoalveolar mission trips. The process of planning a mission includes selecting a population and identifying their unique needs, designing clinic layouts and workflows, team preparation, collection of supplies, fundraising, and advertising. During the mission, methods for protecting privacy, delivering treatment that is standard of care, and sanitation/sterilization options are reviewed. Ethical considerations include avoiding exploitation of vulnerable populations, offending local hosts, need for data collection, and long-term mission sustainability.

Developing a Sustainable Program for Volunteer Surgical Care in Low-Income and Middle-Income Countries   471

Vennila Padmanaban, David Hoffman, Shahid R. Aziz, and Ziad C. Sifri

Volunteer medical missions to low-income and middle-income countries have been a popular but unregulated method of providing care to underserved regions of the world as they work to improve surgical capacity. This article addresses various organizational tenets, such as forming a mission statement, selecting a site location, determining funding sources, establishing a team, patient safety, organization, and postoperative care and follow-up.

The History and Mission of Smile Train, a Global Cleft Charity   481

Angela S. Volk, Matthew J. Davis, Priya Desai, and Larry H. Hollier Jr.

Cleft lip and/or palate (CLP) is a common congenital anomaly with a global impact. One organization attempting to decrease global burden of CLPs is Smile Train. Since

1999, Smile Train has empowered local medical providers to provide comprehensive and sustainable cleft care. Partner surgeons have performed more than 1.5 million operations for patients with CLPs in more than 90 countries. This article outlines the history and mission of Smile Train and details the organization's efforts to increase hospital-wide safety, provide education and training opportunities for partners, and use technology to improve the delivery of cleft care on a global scale.

The success of global outreach surgical programs depends on many factors including the preparation of the surgeons involved in the program. Surgeons in preparing for global outreach programs often focus on surgical procedures or techniques as the most important aspect of the preparation for the program. Just as important to success of the outreach program is the surgeon's familiarity with the language, cultural, and social norms of the host country or region. This article provides valuable information on these issues from three oral and maxillofacial surgeons who have been engaged in global oral and maxillofacial surgery outreach programs for decades.

ORAL AND MAXILLOFACIAL SURGERY CLINICS OF NORTH AMERICA

FORTHCOMING ISSUES

November 2020
Dentoalveolar Surgery
Somsak Sittitavornwong, *Editor*

February 2021
Modern Rhinoplasty and the Management of its Complications
Shahrokh C. Bagheri, Husain Ali Khan, and Behnam Bohluli, *Editors*

May 2021
Advanced Intraoral Surgery
Orrett E. Ogle, *Editor*

RECENT ISSUES

May 2020
Orthodontics for the Craniofacial Surgery Patient
Michael R. Markiewicz, Veerasathpurush Allareddy, and Michael Miloro, *Editors*

February 2020
Orthodontics for the Oral and Maxillofacial Surgery Patient
Michael R. Markiewicz, Veerasathpurush Allareddy, and Michael Miloro, *Editors*

November 2019
Advances in Oral and Maxillofacial Surgery
Jose M. Marchena, Jonathan W. Shum, and Jonathon S. Jundt, *Editors*

SERIES OF RELATED INTEREST

Atlas of the Oral and Maxillofacial Surgery Clinics
www.oralmaxsurgeryatlas.theclinics.com

Dental Clinics
www.dental.theclinics.com

THE CLINICS ARE NOW AVAILABLE ONLINE!
Access your subscription at:
www.theclinics.com

Dedications

This work is dedicated to my late father, Dr Mohammed A. Aziz - a giant in global health, my mother, Dr Fatima B. Aziz, my uncle, Dr M.A. Pasha, MBE, my late aunts, Dr Kamala Pasha and Amina Shariff, my late uncle Akbar Hossain, my rock Teresa Mongelli, Smile Bangladesh board members past and present, all those in Bangladesh and the USA who support Smile Bangladesh, late Smile Bangladesh members - Imre Redai MD and Lynn Speer, and most importantly to my children, Aydin and Samina.

—Shahid R. Aziz

This work is dedicated to my late mother, Mercedes Marchena, an angel with a heart of gold, who taught us the values of authenticity, humility, and generosity, and also to my sister, Marisol, in recognition of her unselfish participation in humanitarian missions, and my dad, Antoninus, for his steady support.

—Jose M. Marchena

I dedicate this edition to my wife, Blythe, my children, Chris, Jennifer, Heather, Meredith, Craig and Melissa. Also Susan Babcock and Susan Clarke-Roser. All have supported me and many participated with me in the global surgery space. And to all who are working toward the goal of safe surgery and anesthesia for all by 2030.

—Steven M. Roser

Shahid R. Aziz, DMD, MD, FACS, FRCS(Ed)
Department of Oral and Maxillofacial Surgery
Rutgers School of Dental Medicine

Division of Plastic Surgery
Department of Surgery
Rutgers–New Jersey Medical School
110 Bergen Street, Room B 854
Newark, NJ 07103, USA

Jose M. Marchena, DMD, MD, FACS
Department of Oral and Maxillofacial Surgery
University of Texas Health Science
Center at Houston
6560 Fannin Street, Suite 1900
Houston, TX 77054, USA

Steven M. Roser, DMD, MD, FACS, FRCS(Ed)
Delos Hill Chair and Professor of Surgery
Chief, Division of Oral and Maxillofacial Surgery
Department of Surgery
Emory University School of Medicine
1365B Clifton Road
Suite 2300
Atlanta, GA 30322, USA

E-mail addresses:
azizsr@sdm.rutgers.edu (S.R. Aziz)
jose.m.marchena@uth.tmc.edu (J.M. Marchena)
sroser@emory.edu (S.M. Roser)

Oral Maxillofacial Surg Clin N Am 32 (2020) xiii
https://doi.org/10.1016/j.coms.2020.05.004
1042-3699/20/© 2020 Published by Elsevier Inc.

Dedications

Preface

Global Oral and Maxillofacial Surgery: The Evolution of a Surgical Specialty Worldwide

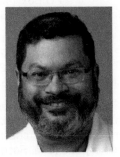
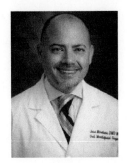
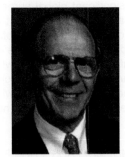

Shahid R. Aziz, DMD, MD, FACS, FRCS(Ed)

Jose M. Marchena, DMD, MD, FACS

Steven M. Roser, DMD, MD, FACS, FRCS(Ed)

Editors

It is a great honor to be guest editors for this unique issue of the *Oral and Maxillofacial Surgery Clinics of North America* on Global Oral and Maxillofacial Surgery.

The Lancet Commission[1] defines global surgery as:

> "An area of study, research, practice, and advocacy that seeks to improve health outcomes and achieve health equity for all people who need surgical and anaesthesia care, with a special emphasis on underserved populations and populations in crisis. It uses collaborative, cross-sectoral, and transnational approaches and is a synthesis of population-based strategies with individual surgical and anesthesia care."

Global surgery has evolved into a major clinical interest among a large group of health care providers, especially surgical trainees who are expressing a desire to participate in global health care opportunities. In a recent survey of oral and maxillofacial surgical residents who participated in surgical missions to Bangladesh, 97% stated it was one of the highlights of their training.[2] Over the last decade, we have witnessed the emergence of formal training programs for humanitarian international surgeons in a variety of surgical specialties. On the other side, surgeons in low income countries are passionate to learn from their international colleagues. Global surgery is not just about providing access to and equity in quality surgical and anesthetic care in the developing world. It also fosters a spirit of unifying humanity through surgery: exchanging ideas with colleagues from different global and socioeconomic countries, training one another and learning from one another.

Although there is a reasonable amount of literature on global surgery in other surgical disciplines, there is little work shared in connection with oral

Oral Maxillofacial Surg Clin N Am 32 (2020) xv–xvi
https://doi.org/10.1016/j.coms.2020.05.002
1042-3699/20/© 2020 Published by Elsevier Inc.

and maxillofacial surgery. It was our intent to collect and to disseminate practical information concerning all aspects of international humanitarian oral and maxillofacial surgery in a single organized publication. The editors and section authors involved in this project, the very first organized publication in global oral and maxillofacial surgery, have all demonstrated a passion for global health and have significant global surgery experience in different areas of the world. It is our hope that this issue of the *Oral and Maxillofacial Surgery Clinics of North America* will serve as a source of practical information for those who are experienced in humanitarian surgical missions as well as for oral and maxillofacial surgeons who are just becoming interested in international humanitarian work.

Shahid R. Aziz, DMD, MD, FACS, FRCS(Ed)
Department of Oral and Maxillofacial Surgery
Rutgers School of Dental Medicine
110 Bergen Street, Room B854
Newark, NJ 07103, USA

Jose M. Marchena, DMD, MD, FACS
Department of Oral and Maxillofacial Surgery
University of Texas Health Science Center at Houston
6560 Fannin Street, Suite 1900
Houston, TX 77030, USA

Steven M. Roser, DMD, MD, FACS, FRCS(Ed)
Division of Oral and Maxillofacial Surgery
Department of Surgery
Emory University School of Medicine
1365b Clifton Road
Atlanta, GA 30322, USA

Smile Bangladesh
PO Box 1403
Mountainside, NJ 07092, USA

Healing the Children North East
219 Kent Road, Suite 20
PO BOX 129
New Milford, CT 06776, USA

E-mail addresses:
azizsr@sdm.rutgers.edu (S.R. Aziz)
jose.m.marchena@uth.tmc.edu (J.M. Marchena)
sroser@emory.edu (S.M. Roser)

REFERENCES

1. Meara J, Leather AJ, Hagander L, et al. Global surgery 2030: evidence and solutions for achieving health, welfare, and economic development. Lancet 2015;386:569–624.
2. Aziz SR, Ziccardi VB, Chuang SK. Survey of residents who have participated in humanitarian medical missions. J Oral Maxillofacial Surg 2012;70(2):e147–57.

Introduction
Global Oral and Maxillofacial Surgery

On September 5, 2002, the CEO of Merck, global health officials, and government officials from East Africa, gathered at Bombani village in the Tanga Region of Tanzania to mark 250 million doses of Mectizan having been given in Africa. This drug, manufactured and donated free by Merck, was used to combat Onchocerciasis, also known as river blindness, to prevent the loss of vision that had marked the lives of millions of Africans over generations. Globalization has often been condemned for its many shortcomings, but I was watching a miracle of globalization. More than that, we are familiar with the idea that if something can go wrong it will go wrong, but here we witnessed the result of so many things going right.

Mectizan came from an unusual place. It was developed from a soil sample taken from a golf course in Japan. It was worked on in a US lab at the Merck Drug Company, where a drug was developed by Merck scientist, William Campbell, to prevent heartworm in dogs. Merck's Senior Director of Clinical Research, the late Dr Mohammad Aziz, who spent years working for the World Health Organization in sub-Saharan Africa, suggested Mectizan could treat and prevent river blindness (**Fig. 1**). To test his hypothesis, Merck CEO P. Roy Vagelos sent Aziz to Senegal, western Africa.

Aziz's clinical trials proved that the drug could prevent blindness due to Onchocerca if given to villagers once a year, indeed a miracle drug.

But the miracle continued. An inexpensive drug, given only once a year to some of the poorest people in the world, was not a lucrative proposition. At the request of Aziz, Campbell, and Vagelos, Merck created the Mectizan Donation Program, donating the drug for free to the developing world. Hundreds of government and nongovernment agencies in Africa became involved, and the World Bank developed a fund to help distribute the drug. Villagers became involved in record keeping and drug distribution. The benefits of medical science were made available to villages, even those that lacked other health facilities. And blindness rates dramatically declined. By 2017, the one-billionth free dose of Mectizan had been delivered, and river blindness, at one time the third leading cause of tropical blindness globally, was all but eradicated in the developing world. This is indeed one of the greatest global public health success stories in history. William Campbell won the 2015 Nobel Prize for his work in developing this drug. Had the Nobel been awarded posthumously, Aziz certainly would have shared it with Campbell.

This is the positive side of globalization.

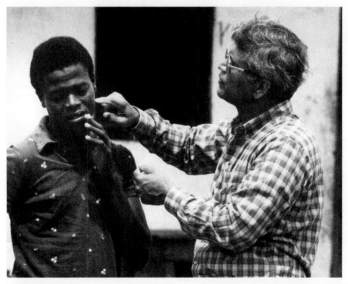

Fig 1. Dr Mohammed Aziz evaluating a young man with river blindness Dakar, Senegal, 1982. While many were involved in the subsequent development and donation of Ivermectin to treat Onchocerciasis, Aziz may have been the key, proving Ivermectin's human application.

Oral Maxillofacial Surg Clin N Am 32 (2020) xvii–xviii
https://doi.org/10.1016/j.coms.2020.05.003
1042-3699/20/© 2020 Published by Elsevier Inc.

And now the son of Mohammad Aziz, Shahid R. Aziz, with colleagues Steven Roser and Jose Marchena, is promoting the idea that oral and maxillofacial surgery, as practiced in rich countries, could benefit all countries as another positive example of globalization.

For decades, skilled surgeons in affluent nations have provided periodic benefits for eye surgery and correction of cleft palates in other countries. In many cases, this expertise has now developed within those countries. India has developed its own world-class expertise in eye and cleft surgery, for example.

But there is much more to offer. Mozambique has trained rural health workers to provide C-sections for women who would otherwise be unable to reach a hospital. What could actually be provided in surgical care at rural health clinics if the same attention could be given to the skills, equipment, and training required for some surgical procedures, similar to the attention that has been given to when and how to treat for pneumonia, dehydration, gastrointestinal problems, plus decision trees to provide guidance on when to send the patient to a hospital?

What might be possible if the surgical experience of industrial countries could be brought to bear on one of the most crippling conditions known, namely, that of fistulas that condemn women to a lifetime of rejection by their families and communities.

What could result from surveillance systems for surgical conditions that are as good as infectious disease surveillance systems? What would happen if oral and maxillofacial surgeons globally succeeded in having a comprehensive program at the World Health Organization that defined oral and facial surgical problems of the world and helped to organize interested professionals in meeting those challenges?

This issue of the *Oral and Maxillofacial Surgery Clinics of North America*, dedicated to global surgery, could be the beginning of a new global oral and maxillofacial surgical renaissance.

William Foege, MD, MPH
Rollins School of Public Health
Emory University
Centers for Disease Control
The Carter Center
Claudia Nance Rollins Building
1518 Clifton Road, CNR 7040H
Atlanta, GA 30322, USA

E-mail address:
Wfoege@emory.edu

Oral and Maxillofacial Surgery

An Opportunity to Improve Surgical Care and Advance Sustainable Development Globally

Ché L. Reddy, MBChB, MPH[a,b,*,1], Rolvix H. Patterson, MD, MPH[a,c,1],
Isaac Wasserman, MD, MPH[a,d], John G. Meara, MD, DMD, MBA[a,b],
Salim Afshar, MD, DMD[a,b,e,*]

KEYWORDS

- Global health • Global surgery • Global health policy • Health systems
- Oral and maxillofacial surgery • Global oral and maxillofacial surgery • Craniofacial surgery
- Oral surgery

KEY POINTS

- Global health has evolved to prioritize frameworks, policy, and interventions that support strengthening health systems to reduce systemic inequity.
- The growing field of global surgery has aligned with these goals and aims to improve access to safe, timely, and affordable surgical care by advancing surgical care within health systems.
- As a surgical subspecialty, oral and maxillofacial surgery has a vital role in reducing the burden of oral and craniofacial conditions through research, advocacy, policy, and practice.

INTRODUCTION

Despite the historical focus of global health on infectious disease, most health loss is now caused by noncommunicable disease (NCD).[1] Oral disorders are the most prevalent NCD; they affect half of the world's population and contribute substantially to morbidity.[1,2] This global challenge requires a concerted global health response, and oral and maxillofacial surgery (OMFS) has a central role to play in addressing the global burden of oral and craniofacial disorders.

Although many in global health now emphasize a health systems approach to address the diverse causes of poor health outcomes, oral disorders and craniofacial conditions remain underprioritized globally.[3] The global burden of oral health did not improve substantially between 1990 and

[a] Program in Global Surgery and Social Change, Department of Global Health and Social Medicine, Harvard Medical School, 641 Huntington Avenue, Boston, MA 02115, USA; [b] Department of Plastic and Oral Surgery, Boston Children's Hospital, 300 Longwood Ave, Boston, MA 02115, USA; [c] Tufts University School of Medicine, 145 Harrison Ave, Boston, MA 02111, USA; [d] Icahn School of Medicine at Mount Sinai, One Gustave L. Levy Place, New York, NY 10029-6574 USA; [e] Harvard School of Dental Medicine, 188 Longwood Ave, Boston, MA 02115 USA

[1] Cofirst authors.

* Corresponding authors. Department or Plastic and Oral Surgery, Boston Children's Hospital, 300 Longwood Avenue, Hunnewell Building, 1st Floor, Boston, MA 02115.

E-mail addresses: CheLen_Reddy@hms.harvard.edu (C.L.R.); Salim.Afshar@childrens.harvard.edu (S.A.)
Twitter: @CheLenReddy (C.L.R.); @RolvixPatterson (R.H.P.); @WassermanIsaac (I.W.); @JohnMeara (J.G.M.); @SalimAfshar (S.A.)

Oral Maxillofacial Surg Clin N Am 32 (2020) 339–354
https://doi.org/10.1016/j.coms.2020.03.001
1042-3699/20/© 2020 Elsevier Inc. All rights reserved.

2015,[4] which highlights the need to ensure comprehensive care for oral disorders and craniofacial conditions. Prevention is essential but, even with strong prevention programs, there will be inevitable cases that require surgical treatment. There is an important advocacy, capacity-building, and policy-shaping role for oral and maxillofacial (OMF) surgeons to support the global health community to reduce the burden of oral disorders through stronger health care systems and universal health coverage (UHC) (**Table 1** provides a glossary of key terms and acronyms).

Historically, surgeons have worked to improve health abroad, predominantly through international surgical trips that focus on well-demarcated areas and populations that are affected by specific clinical conditions. However, it is increasingly recognized that the world is becoming a global, interdependent society in which the health of populations is not predicated on the borders of nation-states.[5,6] This global perspective and the understanding of the benefits of investing in stronger health systems have catalyzed a paradigm shift in global health care toward identifying more sustainable, inclusive, and holistic solutions.

The global health community's perspective on addressing health disparities has evolved from implementing isolated so-called vertical programs, such as stand-alone vaccine delivery or malnutrition screening, to prioritizing support for building quality horizontal health systems.[7] This approach aligns efforts with UHC and international goals such as the United Nations' (UN) Sustainable Development Goals (SDGs), which are 17 objectives to be achieved by the year 2030.[8] SDG 3, which focuses on health, is intended to "ensure healthy lives and promote wellbeing for all at all ages," and 3.4 specifically describes ending premature deaths from NCDs.[9] Surgical care is mostly omitted from global health despite its ability to address many NCDs, including oral disorders.[10,11]

OMFS is necessary to provide comprehensive surgical care through UHC and establish more responsive health systems. However, the role of OMFS in addressing the global burden of surgical disease has not been defined. This article describes the transitioning global health landscape as it relates to surgery, and it outlines how OMFS can support and improve global health care delivery and global health policy to achieve greater equity in health.

Modern History of Global Health

Global health is an area of study and mode of development that has evolved substantially in the modern era. Scholars describe various phases of global health,[12–15] the origins of which are sometimes traced to the colonial era, involve a series of defining changes, and involve a range of people, institutions, activities, themes, and values that make up global health in the present day. The progression of global health through these periods has closely followed global politics[13,16] (the influence of hegemonic powers, and dominant political values), which continue to shape the discourse around health, and what health issues are recognized, valued, and addressed. What is global health? A discipline? A global effort within a broader movement toward sustainable development? An ethos? A value system? A unified and commonly accepted definition is challenging precisely because global health encompasses all of these, is viewed differently by a diverse set of people, and institutions, and is continually evolving. Richard Horton, editor-in-chief of The Lancet, and global health activist, once said of global health: "[It] is an attitude. It is a way of looking at the world. It is about the universal nature of our human predicament. It is a statement about our commitment to health as a fundamental quality of liberty and equity."[12] However, global health is also more than an attitude. It is "a collection of (biosocial) problems, rather than a discipline" for Paul Farmer,[12] cofounder of the nongovernmental organization Partners in Health, and Harvard Medical School Professor in Infectious Diseases and Medical Anthropology. "Problems ranging from epidemics (from AIDS [acquired immunodeficiency syndrome] to polio to noncommunicable diseases) and the development of new technologies (preventative, diagnostic, therapeutic) to the effective delivery of these technologies to those most in need – all turn on the quest for equity."[12] To establish global health as a discipline of enquiry, Farmer[12] suggests, will require resocializing disciplines of history, political science, sociology, and anthropology, together with epidemiology, biology, and clinical practice: a true multidisciplinary science with radical alterations in how global health delivery is studied, systematically pursued, and practiced. Farmer[12] thus places particular emphasis on equity and recognizes the need to draw from a range of clinical and social science disciplines to provide such health care services globally. Global health is not limited to health inequities in low-income and middle-income countries (LMICs); instead, "global health is about health equity everywhere,"[13] including the health disparities in high-income countries and valuing the health of marginalized communities in all parts of the world.

Table 1
Glossary of key terms and acronyms

Term	Definitions
DALYs	"One DALY can be thought of as one lost year of "healthy" life. … DALYs for a disease or health condition are calculated as the sum of the Years of Life Lost (YLL) due to premature mortality in the population and the Years Lost due to Disability (YLD) for people living with the health condition or its consequences."[55]
GBD	"The Global Burden of Disease Study (GBD) is the most comprehensive worldwide observational epidemiological study to date. It describes mortality and morbidity from major diseases, injuries, and risk factors to health at global, national, and regional levels. Examining trends from 1990 to the present and making comparisons across populations enables understanding of the changing health challenges facing people across the world in the 21st century."[56]
GlobalSurg Collaborative	The GlobalSurg Collaborative conducts "collaborative international research into surgical outcomes by fostering local, national, and international research networks."[57]
HICs	Countries classified as high income by the World Bank Country and Lending Groups criteria (gross national income per capita of at least $12,376)[58]
LCoGS	The LCoGS convened an international team of commissioners, advisors, and collaborators with the goal of "embedding surgery within the global health agenda, catalyzing political change, and defining scalable solutions for the provision of quality surgical and anesthesia care for all."[47,59]
LMICs	Countries classified as low income, lower-middle income, or upper-middle income per capita of $12,375 or less)[58]
MDGs	"The eight Millennium Development Goals (MDGs) – which range from halving extreme poverty to halting the spread of HIV/AIDS and providing universal primary education, all by the target date of 2015 – [formed] a blueprint agreed to by all the world's countries and all the world's leading development institutions."[60]
NSOAP	"Driven by the national government and supporting a wider health strategic plan, a national surgical, obstetric, and anesthesia plan (NSOAP) identifies the current gaps in health care, prioritizes solutions, and provides an implementation framework, monitoring, and evaluation plan, and projected cost. The NSOAP establishes a unified vision for the strengthening of surgical systems and coordination of efforts required to achieve this."[61]
Primary health care	"Primary health care is a whole-of-society approach to health and well-being centered on the needs and preferences of individuals, families, and communities. It addresses the broader determinants of health and focuses on the comprehensive and interrelated aspects of physical, mental, and social health and wellbeing."[62]
SADC	An intergovernmental organization consisting of 16 member states that aims to "achieve development, peace, and security, and economic growth, to alleviate poverty, enhance the standard and quality of life of the peoples of Southern Africa."[63]
SDGs	In 2015, all UN member states adopted 17 goals "as a universal call to action to end poverty, protect the planet and ensure that all people enjoy peace and prosperity by 2030."[8]
UN	Founded in 1945, the UN is an international body made up of 193 member states. Directed by its charter, it addresses a range of issues including "peace and security, climate change, sustainable development, human rights, disarmament, terrorism, humanitarian and health emergencies."[64]

(continued on next page)

Table 1
(continued)

Term	Definitions
UHC	"Ensuring that all people have access to needed health services (including prevention, promotion, treatment, rehabilitation, and palliation) of sufficient quality to be effective while also ensuring that the use of these services does not expose the user the financial hardship."[65]
WPRO	This is 1 of 6 WHO regional offices, and it oversees 37 member states that constitute a population of 1.8 billion people in the Western Pacific region. Its role is to "act as a catalyst and advocate for action at all levels, from local to global, on health issues of public concern" in support of the WHO mission[66]
World Bank Group	A collaborative development bank of 189 member states that consists of 5 organizations with the goals to "end extreme poverty within a generation and boost shared prosperity."[67]
WHA	"The World Health Assembly is the decision-making body of the World Health Organization (WHO). It is attended [annually] by delegations from all WHO Member States and focuses on a specific health agenda prepared by the Executive Board."[68]
WHA Resolution 68.15 (WHA 68.15)	Passed at the 68th WHA in 2015, this resolution urged member states and the WHO to take action to promote the provision of emergency and essential surgical care and anesthesia.[69]
WHO	As the lead agency for international health under the UN, the WHO is made up of 194 member states in 6 regions. It aims to improve health across the world, and it supports progress toward UHC[70]

Abbreviations: DALYs, disability-adjusted life years; GBD, Global Burden of Disease; HICs, high-income countries; LCoGS, Lancet Commission on Global Surgery; LMICs, low-income and middle-income countries; MDGs, Millennium Development Goals; NSOAPs, National Surgical, Obstetric, and Anesthesia Plans; SADC, Southern African Development Community; SDGs, Sustainable Development Goals; UN, United Nations; WHA, World Health Assembly; WHO, World Health Organization; WPRO, Western Pacific Regional Office.

Three broad eras of global health are described: a colonial era[3] characterized by efforts to protect colonists from tropical diseases from indigenous peoples; an era of international health,[12] which occurred mostly during the cold war, defined by national health reforms in proxy countries to control the spread of epidemics; and the current modern era characterized by the professionalization of global health, in which there has been a significant increase in research, global health training programs, and global health capacity-building projects.[13] Some may distinguish between 2 phases in the last category: an initial phase dominated by researchers from high-income countries leading research programs in LMICs, and another phase in which LMIC researchers lead programs in LMICs.[13] All of these phases correspond with defining political moments in the history of the modern world: the European colonial conquest; postcolonial independence struggles and the cold war; and the current era, which focuses on global sustainable development.

Global health has progressed in content, values, methods, and actors as it evolved through the 3 eras (**Table 2**). Each era is not neatly bound, finite, or independent. Instead, they are all relational, interactive, and codependent. Methods of inquiry, once dominant in the colonial era, may also be used in the modern, more academic orientation of global health. Progressive values that characterize the modern era of global health may similarly have been held by individuals and institutions during the internationalist era, planting the initial seed for change. Like all historical modes of analysis, attempts to carve out and characterize epochs, or time periods, are limited by how history is told, and who tells that history.[17] Classifications such as these must be interpreted with that awareness and sensitivity; that characterizations constitute broad representations, and more often reflect the dominant narrative rather than the oppressed (or subaltern) experience. Global health efforts during European settler colonialism were defined by values of imperial conquest and domination. The primary objective for settler communities and colonial institutions was political and economic stability; health was approached within that context and was used to protect settler communities and sometimes promote sickness and disease within indigenous populations to advance political and economic objectives. However, the core value in global health has radically changed. Emphasis is now placed on greater equity in health care delivery, based on respecting the universal value of the highest attainable standard of health for all people.[18] Over a period of roughly 4 centuries, the dominant value system in global health has radically changed.

Changes in the values of global health have similarly produced changes in institutions and in what types of work they pursue, and how. From a parochial and conservative group of colonists and settler institutions defining global health efforts during the colonial era, modern global health involves a plurality of institutions (**Table 3**): nation-states, multilateral organizations (eg, World Health Organization [WHO]), academic institutions,

Table 2
An analytical and conceptual framework of the eras of global health

	Values	Content	Methods	Actors
Colonial	Colonial domination and settler hegemony	Protection of colonists from diseases affecting indigenous people	Mostly qualitative studies: anthropologic studies involving of observation of indigenous groups	Elite groups linked to the colonial project
International Health	Realism (international relations)	Vertical health programs designed to prevent the spread of epidemics and maintain health security	Transitioning from methods in the colonial era to the wide range used in the modern era	Nation-states, the emergence of global actors (WHO)
Modern, Professionalized	Equity	Horizontal system-wide interventions for sustainable development	A combination of qualitative and quantitative methods	Plurality of actors

Table 3
Summary of the actors in global health

	Function	Examples
Nation-states	Health policy formation, implementation of legislated health policy, health care provision	All sovereign nations of the world
Multilateral Organizations	Normative frameworks, global governance, and coordination; dissemination of best practice	WHO
Academic Institutions	Research, training, health care provision (academic medical centers)	Global health/policy departments, centers, and programs in the university setting
Bilateral Organizations	Funding and technical assistance	USAID, KOICA
Philanthropy and Foundations	Funding	BMGF, Rockefeller
Development Banks and Innovative Financing Mechanisms	Funding	World Bank Group, Global Fund, GAVI
Private Sector	Health care provision, funding, insurance, disruption	Narayana Health
Nongovernmental Organizations	Health care provision, research, advocacy	MSF, Global Health Policy Center (Center for Strategic and International Studies), PATH, John Snow
Civil Society Organizations	Advocacy, health care provision	TAC

Abbreviations: BMGF, Bill & Melinda Gates Foundation; GAVI, Gavi, the Vaccine Alliance; KOICA, Korea International Cooperation Agency; MSF, Médecins Sans Frontières; USAID, TAC, Treatment Action Campaign; US Agency for International Development.

nongovernmental organizations (eg, Médecins Sans Frontières), foundations and philanthropic funders (eg, Rockefeller Foundation), bilateral organizations (eg, US Agency for International Development [USAID]), think tanks (eg, Center for Strategic and International Studies), and development banks (eg, the World Bank Group). The plurality of institutions that shape modern global health are adapting to many new trends, challenges, and opportunities that pressure contemporary global health systems. Changes in epidemiology, demography, ecology, and climate, and how the global political economy influences what is possible and feasible in a globalized world, requires an interdisciplinary, well-coordinated, and broad set of actors. Emphasis is placed on strengthening health systems using diagonal approaches that harness the dual benefits of the vertical (single intervention) approaches of the past and the more horizontal efforts that improve health system performance. A variety of scientific methods are now used to systematically study the problems of modern global health and identify promising solutions. The resocializing disciplines that Farmer[12,16] believes are so critical for equity in health care delivery work in unison with the scientific disciplines to provide a rich and informing foundation of knowledge and practice from which to solve current global health challenges. Some of the major themes in global health now include maternal and child health, aging populations, infectious diseases (eg, tuberculosis, human immunodeficiency virus [HIV]/AIDS), the financing and governance of health systems, global health security, and the effects of environmental change on population health.

Shifts in global norms about the role of health in human flourishing led to both a rights-based and international development discourse, which has increased the global importance of health for sustainable development. The formation of the UN system in 1945, following the Second World War, and its guiding document, the Universal Declaration of Human Rights (UDHR),[19] for the first time in human history explicitly embraced and respected the value of all human beings in international law within a formalized institutional framework. The UDHR outlines inalienable and universal rights that all people should have respected, including health. In 1948, the WHO was established as a specialized agency of the UN Economic and Social Council to build on and extend the role of health within this formalized institutional framework of the UN. The overall objective of the WHO is to advance the "highest possible attainment of health for all people."[18] The WHO provides an important coordinating function in terms of global governance toward this objective. Special multilateral treaties signed by nation-states within international law have also increased the salience of health as a responsibility of governments to provide to citizens. The International Covenant on Economic, Social, and Cultural Rights (IESCR)[20] is a treaty signed by 71 nation-states that respects specific rights necessary for economic, social, and cultural well-being and was adopted by the UN General Assembly in 1966. The IESCR explicitly mentions the role of health toward this end. Together with the International Covenant on Civil and Political Rights, which deals with protection from the state, rather than the state's responsibility to provide these services to its people, it is part of the UN International Bill on Human Rights.

The global health community has built on these global frameworks to develop, extend, and deepen global public health efforts. The Alma Ata conference of 1978 was a milestone event in public health. It emphasized the importance of primary health care to increase population health worldwide. The Alma Ata Declaration,[21] the consensus document of the conference, was revolutionary and groundbreaking: "Primary health care is essential health care based on practical, scientifically sound, and socially acceptable methods and technology made universally accessible to individuals and families in the community through their full participation and at a cost that the community and country can afford to maintain at every stage of their development in the spirit of self-reliance and self-determination." This unifying definition of primary health care recognizes the value of citizens in the decision making of their health care needs, and of the broader processes of national development, on their own terms: the provision of health care in addressing disparities exists within this transformative context. Most recently, at the UN High-Level Meeting on UHC in New York City, the global development community ratified a renewed commitment for UHC,[22] further emphasizing the critical importance of global health equity in international development, and global peace and security: the core goals of the UN. In addition, global goals for international development have recognized the indispensable role of health. The Millennium Development Goals (MDGs), passed in 2000, focused heavily on maternal and child health (MCH) and HIV. The SDGs (SDG 3 pertains to global health), launched in 2015, focus on health systems strengthening and UHC, in addition to the MCH and HIV priority areas of the MDGs.[23]

In addition to changes at the global level, at the national level, citizens and civil society have become increasingly vocal about their health needs.[24–26] People all over the world care more about their health, and they want health systems that provide quality and affordable health care services. As a result, health is a core issue in most electoral processes as governments try to respond to the health expectations of the citizenry. In high-income and LMICs alike, access to quality, safe, and affordable health care services is of principal importance. Entering the modern era of global health, and in helping to achieve UHC and support SDG attainment, the defining feature of global health will be to engage in all efforts (in a multisectoral and collaborative manner) that collectively achieve this end goal: equity and convergence[27] in health worldwide.

THE EMERGING ROLE OF GLOBAL SURGERY IN THE GLOBAL HEALTH NARRATIVE

As clinicians, epidemiologists, and politicians increasingly looked beyond their borders to promote global health, surgery emerged as a neglected but essential part of the growing toolbox. Although some might worry that surgery represents an inefficient use of resources and infrastructure and an intervention that was resistant to easy and quick fixes, those involved in the promotion of health began advocating for the inclusion of surgery.

As Director-General of the WHO, Halfdan Mahler saw firsthand the need for surgery. Halfway through his term, Dr Mahler[28] devoted an entire speech, "Surgery, and Health for All," to linking surgery to the provision of primary health care. Referencing the 1978 Alma Ata declaration on primary health care, Dr Mahler asserts, "Surgery clearly has an important role to play in primary health care ... yet the vast majority of the world's population has no access whatsoever to skilled surgical care." Moreover, he argues that something unique and special is needed to overcome this problem. "Conventional solutions are not likely to be very satisfactory," Dr Mahler laments. "The number of surgeons involved and the length of their conventional training makes these solutions impractical." Dr Mahler puts this most difficult of global health problems forward, ending with an urgent moral appeal: "I beg of you to give serious consideration to this most serious manifestation of social inequity in health care." However, nearly 30 years after Dr Mahler's 1980 speech, momentum was still lacking for global surgery writ large.

In their attempt to reenergize the global surgery movement, Farmer and Kim[10] in 2008 described surgery as the "neglected stepchild of global public health." They presented a situation in which "within poor countries, surgical services are concentrated almost wholly in cities and reserved largely for those who can pay for them." They even cited how "congenital abnormalities such as cleft palate remain life-long afflictions rather than pediatric surgical disease." They went on to identify the nontransmissible nature of surgical disease as one of the drivers that have prevented surgery being considered a "public problem necessitating public support." Importantly, the carriers of this message must be the surgeons themselves, who must "involv[e] themselves ... to speak fluently about rebuilding infrastructure, training personnel, and delivering high-quality care to the very poorest." They referenced surgical mission trips, and, although acknowledging their role, Drs Farmer and Kim[10] pushed farther, asserting that "donor hospitals, surgeons, and all those involved in efforts to redistribute surgical supplies need to do due diligence and rate their partner institutions in new ways ... do not merely ask about the size and quality of the operating rooms. Ask about your partners' commitment to reaching the poorest." However, there is still a role for surgical missions. "Although we and many others have argued that primary health care, requiring a sustained investment of time and resources, cannot be delivered effectively through such missions, this critique does not always hold true for certain surgical subspecialties. Witness the success of what might be termed 'vertical' surgical missions focusing on a single pathology, such as cleft palate."[10] Thus, the areas for OMF surgeons to participate in and lead global surgery efforts extend to both surgical mission and longer-term capacity-building efforts.

As attention, understanding, and drive built for the inclusion of surgery in the global health movement, surgery was included in 2015 as an official priority for global health. The Disease Control Priorities Network (DCPN), a Gates Foundation project housed at the University of Washington, focuses on strengthening the capacity of evidence-based decision making. Beginning in 2015, they published the third edition of *Disease Control Priorities* (DCP3), a review of the evidence behind cost-effective interventions to address the burden of disease in LMICs. For the first time, DCP dedicated an entire volume (as part of a 9-volume series) to surgery. Previously mentioned in DCP1 and then occupying a chapter in DCP2, the authors of DCP have been acknowledging the importance of surgery in global health. In it, they show "the very large health burden from conditions that are primarily or extensively treated by surgery ... dispel[ling] the myth that surgery is too expensive by showing that many essential surgical services rank amongst the most cost-effective of all health interventions."[29] Congenital anomalies such as cleft lip and palate, in particular, receive particular emphasis, advocating that they be treated at first-level, second-level, and third-level hospitals in an ideal health system.

The Lancet Commission on Global Surgery (LCoGS) published its report, *Global Surgery 2030: Evidence and Solutions for Achieving Health, Welfare, and Economic Development.*[12] Arising from 11 different meetings with collaborators from 110 countries, the report identified 5 key messages for health policymakers:

1. Five billion people lack access to safe, affordable surgical and anesthesia care when needed.
2. One-hundred and forty-three million additional surgical procedures are needed annually.
3. Thirty-three million individuals annually face catastrophic health expenditure because of payment for surgery and anesthesia. An additional 48 million cases of catastrophic expenditure are attributable to the nonmedical costs of accessing surgical care.
4. Investment in surgical and anesthesia services is affordable, saves lives, and promotes economic growth (**Fig. 1**).
5. Surgery is an indivisible, indispensable part of health care.

To end a monumental year in global surgery, the World Health Assembly (WHA) at their 68th meeting made strengthening emergency and essential surgical care and anesthesia a component of UHC. This vital resolution, WHA 68.15, mandated the WHO and the member states to take action toward the development of emergency and essential surgical and anesthesia care. Since then, the current WHO Director-General, Dr Tedros Adhanom Ghebreyesus, proclaimed, "No country can achieve Universal Health Coverage unless its people have access to safe, timely, and affordable surgical services ... It is, therefore, vital that countries invest in surgery."[30]

ORAL AND MAXILLOFACIAL SURGERY IN GLOBAL SURGERY
Burden and Distribution of Oral and Maxillofacial Disease

Oral disease is estimated to affect more than 4 billion people annually, and those of lower socioeconomic status are disproportionately affected.[2,31] Of these, 2.8 billion people have dental caries, 268 million have edentulism and severe tooth decay, and 796 million have periodontal disease.[2] Treatment of these disorders is often within the purview of a dentist. However, OMF surgeons are often needed to address complications of dental disease, infections, benign maxillofacial cysts, tumors and malformations, oral cavity cancer, orofacial clefts, and OMF trauma, among other conditions.

Benign Disorders

OMF conditions need not be malignant to exert a terrible toll on patients. Although data on prevalence and burden (clinical, social, and economic) are not well reported across many countries, particularly in LMICs, they nonetheless likely play an important part in the variety of conditions treated by OMF surgeons. Despite not being malignant, the effects on individuals and their positions in society can be devastating. In addition to facial disfigurement that can cause social isolation, benign disorders often progress because of lack of access to care, resulting in severe functional limitations.

Oral Cavity Cancer

Oral cavity cancer causes substantial morbidity and mortality across the world. In 2017, an estimated

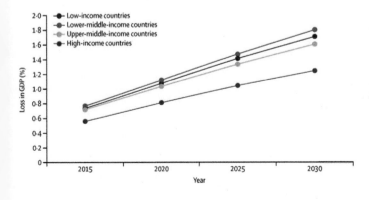

Fig. 1. Annual value of lost economic output caused by surgical conditions. GDP, gross domestic product. (*From* Meara JG, Leather AJM, Hagander L, et al. Global Surgery 2030: evidence and solutions for achieving health, welfare, and economic development. Lancet 2015;386:569–624; with permission.)

1.6 million cases of oral cavity cancer led to 5.3 million disability-adjusted life years (DALYs) and 193,696 deaths.[1,2] Because of mortality alone, it has been estimated that oral cavity cancers will cause $166 billion USD in macroeconomic loss by 2030 (**Fig. 2**). This sum represents 31% of the total head and neck cancer macroeconomic burden, and these losses are greater than that of any other type of head and neck cancer. This burden is unequally distributed, particularly in the South Asia and Southeast Asia, East Asia, and Oceania regions, as defined by the Global Burden of Disease (GBD) study, which will have the most deaths, DALYs, and macroeconomic losses.[1,32] First-line therapy for oral cavity neoplasms is surgical resection, a procedure performed by OMF surgeons.

Orofacial Clefts

GBD 2017 estimates that 10.8 million people have orofacial clefts,[2] which have an extensive impact on quality of life; 652,083 DALYs were attributed to this condition.[1] Untreated orofacial clefts can have lifelong consequences on psychosocial health because of stigma.[33] However, orofacial clefts are treatable by OMF surgeons. Economic benefits of orofacial cleft surgery are estimated to cost $29 to 73 per DALY (**Fig. 3**), which are comparable in terms of cost-effectiveness with widely accepted global health interventions such as

vaccines and medical therapy for ischemic heart disease and HIV/AIDS.[34–36]

Oral and Maxillofacial Trauma

OMF surgeons are well equipped to manage both dental and maxillofacial trauma, given their expertise in both dental and craniofacial surgery. Craniofacial trauma is the cause of approximately half of the estimated total 8.5 million trauma deaths worldwide,[37] and maxillofacial fractures can cause morbidity in the form of aesthetic abnormalities, loss of oral function, and substantial cost to society.[19,20] Existing data on the global epidemiology of craniofacial trauma are sparse; studies typically report craniofacial trauma epidemiology at individual clinical sites. However, the presentation of maxillofacial fracture has been shown to vary by region, and it has been suggested that these variations in trauma often correspond with a country's level of economic development.[38]

More than 1 billion people are estimated to have experienced dental trauma, placing it as the fifth most prevalent disease or injury compared with GBD conditions.[39,40] Despite its ubiquity, dental trauma is widely underreported internationally.[40] Thus, dental trauma care remains expensive and likely out of reach for lower socioeconomic strata.[41] Given the negative social and emotional ramifications of untreated dental trauma, the lack

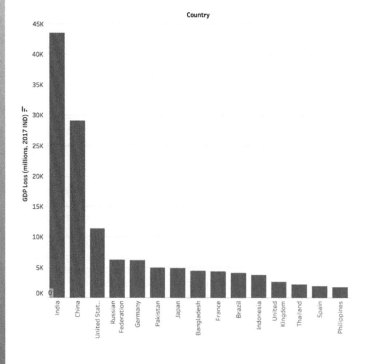

Fig. 2. GDP losses to oral cavity cancer by country 2018 to 2030. IND, International Dollars. (*Data from* Patterson R, Fischman V, Wasserman I, et al. Global burden of head and neck cancer: economic consequences, health, and the role of surgery. Otolaryngol Head Neck Surg. 2020;162(3):296–303.)

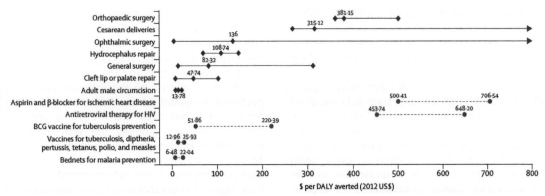

Fig. 3. Annual value of lost economic output in US dollars per DALY averted because of surgical conditions. BCG, bacillus Calmette-Guérin. (*From* Chao TE, Sharma K, Mandigo M, et al. Cost-effectiveness of surgery and its policy implications for global health: a systematic review and analysis. Lancet Glob Health. 2014;2(6):e334-45; with permission.)

of attention to dental trauma likely perpetuates disparities in quality of life.[40]

Noma

Noma, the Greek word for devour, is a necrotizing disease of the face that affects children aged 2 to 6 years who have malnutrition, and it carries a mortality of 90%.[42–44] According to the WHO, noma has an estimated incidence of 140,000 cases per year.[45] Most cases occur within the so-called Noma belt located south of the Saharan desert.[46] Although medical treatment, including intravenous fluids, nutrition, and wound care, can decrease the noma mortality to 10%, survivors are left with severe orofacial defects.[46] These sequelae frequently require surgical correction to improve oral competence and speech.[4] Complex facial reconstruction often requires the knowledge, expertise, and skills of an OMF surgeon.

Benefits of Oral and Maxillofacial Surgery

By alleviating the burden of these conditions, OMFS can contribute to improved health, welfare, and development. For example, timely, safe, and affordable treatment of pediatric patients offers the potential for lifelong accrual of benefits. Furthermore, treating OMF conditions contributes to improved health overall and allows patients to resume social and economic life. Reducing the impact of dental infections on cardiovascular health, cosmetic deformities on psychological health, or OMF trauma can preserve the ability to speak, eat, and engage socially. However, these benefits are only possible within a functional health care system that delivers OMF health care in a responsive manner through UHC.

Global Oral Health Care Workforce

The health care workforce, including surgical providers, is a pillar of a functional health system,[47] but many health systems across the world are limited by an inadequate workforce. It was estimated that the current global health worker density must grow by 85% in order to meet the 2030 SDGs.[48] This gap profoundly affects the delivery of high-quality oral health care, which requires health workers at all levels of the health system.[37] Primary oral health care is often delivered by dentistry personnel, and surgical oral health care is provided by OMF surgeons.

For dentistry specifically, the WHO reports that more than 93% of member state countries have inadequate numbers of trained workers at less than 1 dentistry worker per 1000 population.[49,50] Globally, workforce planning is limited, and dental workforce planning rarely extends beyond setting a target dentist-population ratio, even in Organisation for Economic Co-operation and Development countries.[51]

The current global surgical workforce is grossly inadequate and inequitably distributed; LMICs are most severely afflicted by surgical workforce shortages.[20] It is likely that OMFS faces the same challenges, but there exist few data on the global OMFS workforce. There is no central repository for OMFS workforce data, only national-level data published for specific countries. There is a pressing need for a comprehensive assessment of the global OMFS workforce.

The specialist surgical workforce indicator collected in the World Bank's World Development Indicators (WDI) represents surgeon, anesthetist, and obstetrician density per 100,000 people. This index attempts to incorporate all surgical subspecialties, including OMFS, and is the only existing representation of the global OMFS workforce. Relevant to OMFS practice, it has been shown that, as the surgical workforce grows, more procedures are done and patients have better head and neck cancer outcomes.[32,47]

Data are further limited on other critical aspects of global OMFS care delivery, such as financial risk protection, infrastructure, training, financing, and what bundled services may comprise an essential OMFS package (in different contexts and scenarios) through UHC. Research on these health system components must be undertaken in order to understand better opportunities to improve OMFS care.

ONGOING STEPS FOR GLOBAL SURGERY

As the global surgery community builds on the momentum arising from the last 2 decades, 3 main areas of focus arise: (1) data and accountability, (2) policy advocacy, and (3) funding mechanisms. The OMFS surgeon and community has a role to play in each of these 3 priorities.

Data and Accountability

Rooted in the maxim that what cannot be measured cannot be managed, the global surgery movement has sought to ground itself in data-driven and evidence-based approaches. These efforts take place at all levels, from multinational organizations to country-specific endeavors. The key to success here is the standardization of relevant indicators, with early sharing and dissemination of data. There are existing efforts to collect high-quality and robust data, but more work is needed to help centralize and standardize these disparate efforts. The WDI were organized by the World Bank, which compiles cross-country comparisons on development indicators pertaining to global health. With more than 1400 time-series indicators for 217 economies (and >40 country groups), the WDI allow for comparative insights that reach back more than 50 years for many indicators. In particular, the WDI contains time-series data collected at regular intervals over a period of time from a wide range of sources, including international organizations, national statistical offices, sample surveys, World Bank country offices, and academia, with disaggregation such as by age, sex, geographic area, or wealth. The World Bank also hosts many databases other than the WDI, such as thematic databases in the DataBank, and collections in the Microdata Library.

More specific to surgery, the African Surgical Outcomes Study (ASOS) was a multicenter 7-day evaluation of patient care and clinical outcomes for patients undergoing surgery in 2016.[52] It ultimately enrolled a prospective cohort of 11,422 patients with 30-day follow-up for a primary outcome of in-hospital postoperative complications in adult surgical patients. Importantly, they found that, "despite a low-risk profile and few postoperative complications, patients in Africa were twice as likely to die after surgery when compared with the global average for postoperative deaths." As

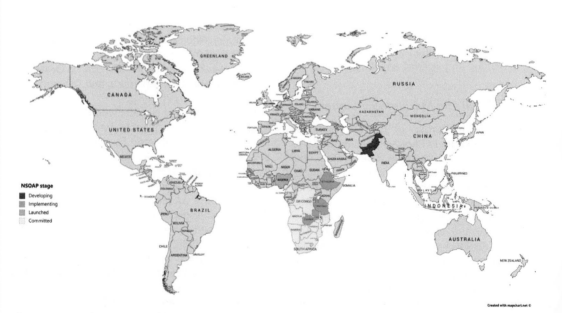

Fig. 4. NSOAP adoption at a global level. (Source: Original data with map template adapted from mapchart.net under CC BY 2.0 license.)

surgeons seek to promote surgical interventions, ASOS reminds the global surgery community that "initiatives to increase access to surgical treatments in Africa should be coupled with improved surveillance for deteriorating physiology in patients who develop postoperative complications."[52]

wArising from these initiatives, the desire to coordinate both a research agenda and projects arose across myriad countries and clinicians. The United Kingdom's National Institute for Health Research Global Research Unit on Global Surgery formed the GlobalSurg initiative in 2017. Although a consortium between the Universities of Birmingham, Edinburgh, and Warwick, GlobalSurg's goal is to represent practicing surgeons around the world to support collaborative research into surgical outcomes. As of their latest round, 5000 clinicians in more than 100 countries are participants.[53]

In a growing effort to help standardize and coordinate research metrics, the Utstein Meeting on Indicators and Reporting Criteria for Surgery, Obstetrics and Anesthesia Patient Safety took place in 2019. Thirty-six experts met to better define indicators and various reporting criteria, with the goal of harmonizing their collection, impact, and comparability.[54]

Policy changes

As reliable and equitable data are collected, those insights can and should be operationalized into policy. OMFS surgeons again have a role to play, in helping to interpret those data for policymakers as well as serving as agenda setters in their own regard.

National Surgical, Obstetric, and Anesthesia Plans (NSOAPs) are the framework advanced by the LCoGS to guide a coordinated, country-level approach to improve access to safe and affordable surgery (**Fig. 4**). NSOAPs emphasize the importance of thoughtful, explicit, and long-term planning across many levels of government in order to achieve better surgical access to citizens in a country. Included in this framework are emergency and trauma surgery, as well as pediatric and oncology surgery (among all other subspecialties). The NSOAP framework centers around 6 domains: infrastructure, service delivery, workforce training, education, information management, financing, and governance (**Fig. 5**). It is intended that NSOAPs are to be integrated within National Strategic Health Plans of countries to ensure that efforts to improve surgery are aligned with the other strategic health priorities of the government (including UHC) and to promote adequate

financing, governance, and coordination for implementation.

Although national-level plans represent a substantial step forward in coordination from the district-level or state-level planning, coordination at a regional (transnational) level is also taking place. Through the Western Pacific Regional Office (WPRO) of the WHO, the Pacific Islands are adopting a regional approach to strengthen surgical care. Emphasis is placed on an integrated and coordinated approach, together with working with regional professional societies such as the Royal Australasian College of Surgeons. These Pacific Islands have also been strong advocates for surgical care within the region, helping to promote the salience of surgery in the WPRO regional health strategy.

In a landmark resolution, 16 member states of the Southern African Development Community signed a regional intergovernmental agreement in November 2018 to reprioritize the provision of surgical care as part of their broader regional health strategy. This resolution represents a special commitment from a regional political entity (comprising both health and finance ministers) to improve surgical care for 300 million people.

WAY FORWARD AND SUMMARY

The discourse around health has evolved to form a critical component of global sustainable

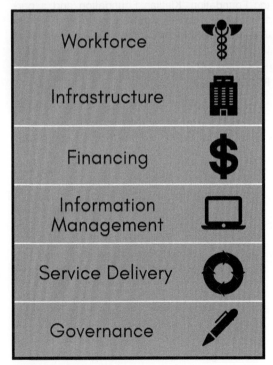

Fig. 5. The NSOAP domains.

development and human social progress. The global health community, initially focusing on primary health care and isolated interventions for specific health conditions, now accepts the importance of stronger health systems and improved global governance and coordination to meet modern health care needs. Surgical care will form an essential aspect of global efforts to achieve UHC. The increasing unmet need for OMFS conditions and the resultant losses in welfare, and sustainable development as a result of failing to invest in OMFS, requires a sustained and concerted effort from the global health community. Such an effort will necessitate systematic study into the nature of OMFS conditions affecting different societies, the distribution of OMFS conditions, and the broader dynamics of how best to provide OMFS health care services through UHC in varied and diverse socioeconomic and cultural contexts. The role of OMF surgeons around the world in helping to achieve this global health priority cannot be overemphasized; there is an extraordinary opportunity to strengthen research, policy, and dialogue as scalable best-practice models are identified to support the achievement of equity in global health, and especially in OMF care.

DISCLOSURE

The Program in Global Surgery and Social Change (PGSSC) receives funding from the General Electric Foundation, Kletjian Foundation and a personal donation from Ronda Stryker and William Johnston. John Meara is the Program Director of the PGSSC.

REFERENCES

1. GBD 2017 DALYs and HALE Collaborators. Global, regional, and national disability-adjusted life-years (DALYs) for 359 diseases and injuries and healthy life expectancy (HALE) for 195 countries and territories, 1990–2017: a systematic analysis for the Global Burden of Disease Study 2017. Lancet 2018;392(10159):1859–922.

2. GBD 2017 Disease and Injury Incidence and Prevalence Collaborators. GBD 2017 Disease and Injury Incidence and Prevalence Collaborators. Global, regional, and national incidence, prevalence, and years lived with disability for 354 diseases and injuries for 195 countries and territories, 1990-2017: a systematic analysis for the Global Burden of Disease Study 2017. Lancet 2018;392(10159): 1789–858.

3. Benzian H, Hobdell M, Holmgren C, et al. Political priority of global oral health: an analysis of reasons for international neglect. Int Dent J 2011;61(3):124–30.

4. Kassebaum NJ, Smith AGC, Bernabé E, et al. Global, regional, and national prevalence, incidence, and disability-adjusted life years for oral conditions for 195 countries, 1990–2015: a systematic analysis for the global burden of diseases, injuries, and risk factors. J Dent Res 2017;96(4):380–7.

5. The Revolution That Global Health Security Needs. JIA SIPA. 2017. Available at: https://jia.sipa.columbia.edu/online-articles/revolution-global-health-security-needs. Accessed February 21, 2019.

6. Haass RN. World order 2.0 2017. Available at: https://www.foreignaffairs.com/articles/2016-12-12/world-order-20. Accessed November 10, 2019.

7. Kruk ME, Gage AD, Arsenault C, et al. High-quality health systems in the Sustainable Development Goals era: time for a revolution. Lancet Glob Health 2018;6(11):e1196–252.

8. United Nations Development Programme. Sustainable Development Goals. UNDP. 2012. Available at: https://www.undp.org/content/undp/en/home/sustainable-development-goals.html. Accessed May 24, 2019.

9. World Health Organization. SDG 3: Ensure healthy lives and promote wellbeing for all at all ages. Available at: http://www.who.int/sdg/targets/en/. Accessed February 20, 2019.

10. Farmer PE, Kim JY. Surgery and global health: a view from beyond the OR. World J Surg 2008; 32(4):533–6.

11. Christie SA, Nwomeh BC, Krishnaswami S, et al. Strengthening surgery strengthens health systems: a new paradigm and potential pathway for horizontal development in low- and middle-income countries. World J Surg 2019;43(3):736–43.

12. Farmer P, editor. Reimagining global health: an introduction. Berkeley (CA): University of California Press; 2013.

13. Abimbola S. On the meaning of global health and the role of global health journals. Int Health 2018; 10(2):63–5.

14. Richard Smith: Moving from global heath 3.0 to global health 4.0 - The BMJ. Available at: https://blogs.bmj.com/bmj/2013/10/08/richard-smith-moving-from-global-heath-3-0-to-global-health-4-0/. Accessed October 1, 2019.

15. Mukherjee J. An introduction to global health delivery: practice, equity, human rights. Oxford: Oxford University Press; 2018.

16. Farmer P. The uses of Haiti. Monroe (ME).: Common Courage Press; 2006.

17. Morris RC, Spivak GC, editors. Can the subaltern speak? reflections on the history of an idea. New York: Columbia University Press; 2010.

18. World Health Organization. World health organization: constitution. 1946. Available at: https://www.who.int/governance/eb/who_constitution_en.pdf. Accessed April 28, 2020.

19. Universal Declaration of Human Rights. United Nations, 217 (III) A, 1948, Paris, art 1. Available at: http://www.un.org/en/universal-declaration-human-rights/. Accessed May 1, 2020.

20. OHCHR | International Covenant on Economic, Social and Cultural Rights. Available at: https://www.ohchr.org/EN/professionalinterest/pages/cescr.aspx. Accessed October 1, 2019.

21. WHO | WHO called to return to the Declaration of Alma-Ata. WHO. Available at: http://www.who.int/social_determinants/tools/multimedia/alma_ata/en/. Accessed November 4, 2019.

22. Universal health coverage political declaration. 2019. Available at: https://www.un.org/pga/73/wp-content/uploads/sites/53/2019/05/UHC-Political-Declaration-zero-draft.pdf. Accessed April 28, 2020.

23. Sustainable Development Goals. UNDP. Available at: https://www.undp.org/content/undp/en/home/sustainable-development-goals.html. Accessed February 19, 2019.

24. Trump campaign views healthcare as a 2020 campaign weapon - Reuters. Available at: https://www.reuters.com/article/us-usa-election-trump/trump-campaign-views-healthcare-as-a-2020-campaign-weapon-idUSKCN1SU12T. Accessed October 1, 2019.

25. Wilkinson E. The NHS: what are the UK's political parties promising? Lancet 2015;385(9973):1059–62.

26. South Africa puts initial universal healthcare cost at $17 billion - Reuters. Available at: https://www.reuters.com/article/us-safrica-health/south-africa-puts-initial-universal-healthcare-cost-at-17-billion-idUSKCN1UY1R2. Accessed October 1, 2019.

27. Jamison DT, Summers LH, Alleyne G, et al. Global health 2035: a world converging within a generation. Lancet 2013;382(9908):1898–955.

28. Mahler H. Surgery and Health for All. Address by Director General of World Health Organization delivered to XXII Biennial World Congress of the International College of Surgeons. Mexico, June 29, 1980. Available at: http://www.who.int/surgery/strategies/Mahler1980speech.pdf?ua=1. Accessed April 27, 2020.

29. Mock CN, Donkor P, Gawande A, et al. Essential surgery: key messages from Disease Control Priorities, 3rd edition. Lancet Lond Engl 2015;385(9983):2209–19.

30. Program in global surgery and social change, Harvard Medical School. WHO Director General Dr. Tedros addressing the global surgery community March 20, 2019. Available at: https://www.youtube.com/watch?v=P1XLthxQs7g. Accessed November 29, 2019.

31. Hobdell MH, Oliveira ER, Bautista R, et al. Oral diseases and socio-economic status (SES). Br Dent J 2003;194(2):91–6.

32. Patterson R, Fischman V, Wasserman I, et al. Global burden of head and neck cancer: economic consequences, health, and the role of surgery. Otolaryngol Head Neck Surg 2020;162(3):296–303.

33. Mzezewa S, Muchemwa FC. Reaction to the birth of a child with cleft lip or cleft palate in Zimbabwe. Trop Doct 2010;40(3):138–40.

34. Corlew DS. Estimation of impact of surgical disease through economic modeling of cleft lip and palate care. World J Surg 2010;34(3):391–6.

35. Gosselin RA, Thind A, Bellardinelli A. Cost/DALY averted in a small hospital in sierra leone: what is the relative contribution of different services? World J Surg 2006;30(4):505–11.

36. Chao TE, Sharma K, Mandigo M, et al. Cost-effectiveness of surgery and its policy implications for global health: a systematic review and analysis. Lancet Glob Health 2014;2(6):e334–45.

37. World Dental Federation. Oral health Atlas 2015. Available at: https://www.fdiworlddental.org/resources/oral-health-atlas/oral-health-atlas-2015. Accessed September 2, 2019.

38. Brasileiro BF, Passeri LA. Epidemiological analysis of maxillofacial fractures in Brazil: A 5-year prospective study. Oral Surg Oral Med Oral Pathol Oral Radiol Endod 2006;102(1):28–34.

39. Petti S, Glendor U, Andersson L. World traumatic dental injury prevalence and incidence, a meta-analysis—One billion living people have had traumatic dental injuries. Dent Traumatol 2018;34(2):71–86.

40. Petti S, Andreasen JO, Glendor U, et al. The fifth most prevalent disease is being neglected by public health organisations. Lancet Glob Health 2018;6(10):e1070.

41. Firmino RT, Siqueira MBLD, Vieira-Andrade RG, et al. Prediction factors for failure to seek treatment following traumatic dental injuries to primary teeth. Braz Oral Res 2014;28(1):1–7.

42. Bourgeois DM, Diallo B, Frieh C, et al. Epidemiology of the incidence of oro-facial noma: a study of cases in Dakar, Senegal, 1981-1993. Am J Trop Med Hyg 1999;61(6):909–13.

43. Tempest MN. Cancrum oris. Br J Surg 1966;53(11):949–69.

44. World Health Organization Regional Office for Africa. Information brochure for early detection and management of noma. 2016. Available at: https://www.afro.who.int/sites/default/files/2017-07/Information_brochure_EN.pdf. Accessed September 02, 2019.

45. Bourgeois DM, Leclercq MH. The World Health Organization initiative on noma. Oral Dis 1999;5(2):172–4.

46. Shaye DA, Winters R, Rabbels J, et al. Noma surgery. Laryngoscope 2019;129(1):96–9.

47. Meara JG, Leather AJM, Hagander L, et al. Global Surgery 2030: evidence and solutions for achieving

health, welfare, and economic development. Lancet 2015;386(9993):569–624.

48. Lancet T. Health-care system staffing: a universal shortfall. Lancet 2018;392(10161):2238.

49. Mathur MR, Williams DM, Reddy KS, et al. Universal Health Coverage. J Dent Res 2015;94(3 Suppl): 3S–5S.

50. World Health Organization. Density of dentistry personnel (total number per 1000 population, latest available year). WHO. Available at: http://www.who.int/gho/health_workforce/dentistry_density_text/en/. Accessed September 2, 2019.

51. Ahern S, Woods N, Kalmus O, et al. Needs-based planning for the oral health workforce - development and application of a simulation model. Hum Resour Health 2019;17. https://doi.org/10.1186/s12960-019-0394-0.

52. Biccard BM, Madiba TE, Kluyts HL, et al. Perioperative patient outcomes in the African Surgical Outcomes Study: a 7-day prospective observational cohort study. Lancet 2018;391(10130):1589–98.

53. Shaw K. About GlobalSurg. Globalsurg. Available at: https://globalsurg.org/who-we-are/. Accessed November 11, 2019.

54. Gore-Booth J, Mellin-Olsen J. Data matters: implications for surgery and anesthesia in achieving universal health coverage. Can J Anesth 2019;66: 143–8.

55. World Health Organization. Metrics: Disability-Adjusted Life Year (DALY). WHO. Available at: https://www.who.int/healthinfo/global_burden_disease/metrics_daly/en/. Accessed November 23, 2019.

56. The Lancet. Global Burden of Disease. Executive Summary. Available at: https://www.thelancet.com/gbd?utm_content=bufferc6c10&utm_medium=social&utm_source=twitter.com&utm_campaign=buffer. Accessed November 23, 2019.

57. NIHR Global Health Research Unit on Global Surgery. About GlobalSurg. Globalsurg. Available at: https://globalsurg.org/who-we-are/. Accessed November 23, 2019.

58. The World Bank Group. World Bank Country and Lending Groups. The World Bank. Available at: https://datahelpdesk.worldbank.org/knowledgebase/articles/906519-world-bank-country-and-lending-groups. Accessed November 23, 2019.

59. The Lancet. The Lancet Commission on global surgery - Executive summary. Available at: https://www.thelancet.com/commissions/global-surgery. Accessed November 23, 2019.

60. United Nations. United Nations Millennium Development Goals. Available at: https://www.un.org/millenniumgoals/bkgd.shtml. Accessed November 23, 2019.

61. Sonderman KA, Citron I, Meara JG. National surgical, obstetric, and anesthesia planning in the context of global surgery: the way forward. JAMA Surg 2018;153(10):959–60.

62. World Health Organization. Primary health care. Available at: https://www.who.int/news-room/fact-sheets/detail/primary-health-care. Accessed November 23, 2019.

63. Southern African development community. SADC Overview. Available at: https://www.sadc.int/about-sadc/overview/. Accessed November 23, 2019.

64. United Nations. About the UN - Overview 2014. Available at: https://www.un.org/en/sections/about-un/overview/index.html. Accessed November 23, 2019.

65. World Health Organization. Universal Health Coverage. WHO. Available at: http://www.who.int/healthsystems/universal_health_coverage/en/. Accessed November 23, 2019.

66. World Health Organization. WHO in the Western Pacific. WPRO. Available at: http://www.wpro.who.int/about/en/. Accessed November 23, 2019.

67. The World Bank Group. About the World Bank. World Bank. Available at: https://www.worldbank.org/en/about. Accessed November 23, 2019.

68. World Health Organization. World Health Assembly. Available at: https://www.who.int/about/governance/world-health-assembly. Accessed November 23, 2019.

69. World Health Assembly. WHA 68.15: Strengthening emergency and essential surgical care and anaesthesia as a component of universal health coverage. 2015. Available at: http://apps.who.int/gb/ebwha/pdf_files/wha68/a68_r15-en.pdf. Accessed December 5, 2018.

70. World Health Organization. WHO brochure. Available at: https://www.who.int/about/what-we-do/who-brochure. Accessed November 23, 2019.

Oral and Maxillofacial Surgery in Low-Income and Middle-Income Countries

Jessica S. Lee, DDS, MD, MA[a], Steven M. Roser, DMD, MD, FRCS(Ed)[b,c,d,e],*,
Shahid R. Aziz, DMD, MD, FRCS(Ed)[f,g,h,i]

KEYWORDS

- Low-income country • Middle-income country • Global oral and maxillofacial surgery

KEY POINTS

- The burden of inadequate access to safe and affordable surgical care falls heaviest on individuals living in low-income and middle-income countries (LMIC).
- Efforts to scale up the global oral and maxillofacial surgery (OMS) workforce to provide quality care must be undertaken by the LMIC in need with assistance from high-income countries.
- The initiation, support, and funding of research on the global burden of oral and maxillofacial surgical conditions to develop a global OMS capacity-building strategy is imperative.

An estimated 5 billion people across the globe do not have access to safe, affordable surgical and anesthesia care.[1] In 2010, there were an estimated 16.9 million deaths from conditions requiring adequate surgical care, representing 32.9% of all deaths worldwide.[2] Over the past 2 decades, global health has mainly focused on the health care solutions for individual, communicable disease such that the deaths related to inadequate access to surgical care have surpassed the number of deaths related to human immunodeficiency virus (HIV)/AIDS (1.46 million), tuberculosis (1.2 million), and malaria (1.17 million) combined.[1,3,4] The burden of inadequate access to safe and affordable surgical care falls heaviest on individuals living in low-income and middle-income countries (LMIC), where 9 out of 10 people do not have access to basic surgical care.[1] As a result, common, easily treatable medical and surgical illnesses become surgical conditions with high morbidity and fatality rates. However, the breadth of surgical disease (eg, infection; cancer; trauma; conditions related to reproductive, maternal, and child health) contributes to the difficulty in the measurement of prevalence and effect of surgical conditions, thus resulting in the surgical burden of adequate care, which contributes to the lagging efforts of establishing surgical and anesthesia care within the epidemiologic, global health framework of disease-based monitoring and advocacy.[1]

In response to these increasing challenges, the Lancet Commission on Global Surgery was launched in January 2014 to examine surgery as an integral component of health care, focusing on LMIC, assessing the challenges and

[a] Pediatric Cleft and Craniofacial Surgery, Cleft and Craniofacial Center, Charleston Area Medical Center Women & Children's Hospital, 830 Pennsylvania Avenue, Suite 302, Charleston, WV 25302, USA; [b] Division of Oral and Maxillofacial Surgery, Department of Surgery, Emory University School of Medicine, 1365B Clifton Road, Atlanta, GA 30322, USA; [c] Healing the Children, Northeast; [d] Committee on Global Surgery, G4 Alliance, International Association of Oral and Maxillofacial Surgery Foundation; [e] Emory Perioperative Global Health Group, Department of Surgery, Emory University School of Medicine; [f] Department of Oral and Maxillofacial Surgery, Rutgers School of Dental Medicine, 110 Bergen Street, Room B854, Newark, NJ 07103, USA; [g] Division of Plastic and Reconstructive Surgery, Department of Surgery, Rutgers - New Jersey Medical School, Newark, NJ, USA; [h] Update Dental College, Dhaka, Bangladesh; [i] Smile Bangladesh
* Corresponding author.
E-mail address: sroser@emory.edu

Oral Maxillofacial Surg Clin N Am 32 (2020) 355–365
https://doi.org/10.1016/j.coms.2020.04.001
1042-3699/20/© 2020 Elsevier Inc. All rights reserved.

opportunities in the development and delivery of quality surgical and anesthesia services in resource-poor settings, and proposing a series of key policy recommendations and indicators to guide future progress.[1]

GLOBAL SURGERY IN LOW-INCOME AND MIDDLE-INCOME COUNTRIES

As an emerging global epidemiologic field, global surgery is defined as "an area of study, research, practice, and advocacy that seeks to improve health outcomes and achieve health equity for all people who need surgical and anesthesia care, with a special emphasis on underserved populations and populations in crisis. It uses collaborative, cross-sectoral, and transnational approaches and is a synthesis of population-based strategies with individual surgical and anesthesia care."[5] The Lancet Commission stratifies the priorities of procedures by volume and risk, focusing on the provision of high-volume, low-risk planned procedures at first-level hospitals and referring the remainder to tertiary facilities.[1] These first-level hospitals should aim to offer a broad range of surgical procedures, with consistent provision of planned surgery requiring only a marginal increase in resources compared with those already in place for emergency care. Because many first-level hospitals in LMIC do not have an option to refer to higher-level, tertiary care centers because of resource and funding constraints, first-level providers should do their best to provide the necessary medical intervention within their facilities. An outline stratifying surgical procedures in a must-do, should-do, and can-do framework was devised to assist in the appropriate prioritization and delegation of procedures in first-level hospitals (**Fig. 1**).[1]

GLOBAL ORAL AND MAXILLOFACIAL SURGERY IN LOW-INCOME AND MIDDLE-INCOME COUNTRIES

Using this framework of the definition provided by the Lancet Commission, global oral and maxillofacial surgery (OMS) can be defined as an area of study, research, practice and advocacy that seeks to improve health outcomes in the evaluation and treatment within OMS, such as infection, dentoalveolar surgery, trauma, cleft and craniofacial anomalies, benign and malignant disorders, and reconstruction to achieve health equity for all people who need oral and maxillofacial surgical and anesthesia care, with a special emphasis on underserved populations and populations in crisis.

Furthermore, surgical procedure stratification into the must-do, should-do, and can-do framework can be adapted in the context of OMS. The management of oral and maxillofacial trauma, dentoalveolar surgery, and infection should be stratified within the must-do framework for first-level hospitals. The management of benign and malignant disorders, reconstruction, temporomandibular joint (TMJ) dysfunction, orthognathic surgery, and cleft and craniofacial anomalies should be stratified under the should-do or can-do framework; the must-do framework for less complex procedures such as small tumor resection with local flap reconstruction and cleft lip/palate, and the should-do or can-do framework for more complex procedures, which may require multidisciplinary specialist support with specialized instruments and hospital units (eg, intensive care unit), including, but not limited to, management of TMJ dysfunction, complex craniofacial anomalies (eg, craniosynostosis), and large head and neck tumor resection with free flap reconstruction.

STRATEGY AND RESOURCE NEEDS FOR SAFE AND EFFECTIVE GLOBAL ORAL AND MAXILLOFACIAL SURGERY

Before the implementation of the specialty of OMS within the framework of global surgery, a needs assessment must be completed to assess the incidence of OMS conditions, the access to providers trained to provide these services, the presence of trained providers, and presence of necessary infrastructure to support these services. This needs assessment can be further refined and adapted based on the setting of the hospital, its scope of practice, and level of care provided by the facility (eg, first vs tertiary). These needs can differ by region (eg, countries) and communities, and assessment of these needs should be undertaken on a global basis by oral and maxillofacial surgeons as a profession. This approach will allow the development of strategies and national surgical plans that include education and training, development of standards of care, implementation of outcome assessment measures, and identification of infrastructure needs based on the LMIC within which the facility operates.

Official investments should be focused on basic needs of delivering surgical and anesthesia care, from electricity and water to radiograph machines and medications, in order to achieve a well-distributed, shared-delivery infrastructure.[6] Although many organizations have characterized specific methods, equipment/instruments, and medication needs for the delivery of surgical and

Must do	Should do	Can do
Acute, high-value procedures that need consistency through local structures; and less complex, urgent procedures that can be delivered through these same structures.	High-priority, high-volume procedures for planned surgery at the first-level hospital.	Important procedures potentially needing specialist support. Ideally, higher-risk procedures should be done at tertiary centres, or done at first-level hospitals with the assistance of visiting super-specialist teams.
Acute, high-value procedures include	Lower-risk procedures include	Examples include
• Laparotomy • Caesarean delivery • Treatment of open fracture	• Hernia repair • Contracture release • Superficial soft tissue tumor resection • Gastroscopy	• Thoracic surgery • Transurethral resection of prostate • Ureterorenoscopy • Vesicovaginal fistula
Lesser complex, urgent procedures include	Medium-risk procedures include	• Basic skin flaps • Rectal prolapse repair
• Wound debridement • Dilation and currettage • Closed fracture reduction	• Cholecystectomy • Intracranial hematoma evacuation • Thyroidectomy • Mastectomy	• Cataract • Cleft lip and palate repair

Fig. 1. Common surgical procedures stratified in a must-do, should-do, and can-do framework for first-level care. (*From* Meara JG, Leather AJM, Hagander L, et al. Global Surgery 2030: evidence and solutions for achieving health, welfare, and economic development. Lancet 2015;386:586; with permission.)

anesthesia care, the endorsement of any specific list should be avoided because needs and the availability of resources within a specific region or country change with time and between contexts.[1] With this in mind, the Lancet Commission has put forth recommendations on the general needs for safe surgery from a review of the existing academic and gray literature and expert panel deliberation, avoiding an overly prescriptive set of recommendations (**Box 1**).[1,7] These 10 needs can be tailored for the implementation of global oral and maxillofacial surgical and anesthetic care, as follows:

1. A trained oral and maxillofacial surgeon, ideally practicing the full scope of OMS, to deliver surgical care
2. An anesthesia provider, ideally trained in delivering anesthesia to children, adults, and patients with complex airway needs caused by head and neck trauma, disorders, and/or congenital anomalies.
3. In addition to basic needs for a hospital (eg, electricity, water, basic laboratory tests, and imaging), specific instruments and supplies to perform safe OMS, with the ability to treat head/neck infections; facial trauma, including fixation of bony structures (eg, fixation plates and screws); dentoalveolar surgery, including management of impacted teeth (eg, surgical handpiece with burs); cleft lip/palate; head/neck disorders (benign and malignant); and general anesthesia with the ability to manage

complex airways secondary to maxillofacial trauma or disorders (eg, video-assisted and/or fiberoptic intubation)
4. Decontamination and sterilization of OMS instruments and general anesthesia equipment
5. Blood supply that is safe and affordable for patients who require transfusions (eg, multisystem trauma, head/neck disorders)
6. Medications, including antibiotics, pain medications, and anesthetics
7. Nursing care tailored to OMS patients both on the floor and intensive care units
8. Twenty-four-hour coverage by oral and maxillofacial surgeons and anesthesiologists in both the emergency department and inpatient units
9. Quality-improvement processes for auditing perioperative morbidity and mortality in the outpatient and inpatient settings
10. Risk assessment and operation planning for emergency and elective oral and maxillofacial surgical procedures

This list can, and should, be adapted based on the needs and availability of resources within a specific region or country.

UNIVERSAL HEALTH COVERAGE FOR GLOBAL ORAL AND MAXILLOFACIAL SURGERY AND ANESTHETIC SERVICES

Out-of-pocket (OOP) payments for health care are the predominant form of financing in many regions,

trillion), particularly in LMIC in southeast Asia, east Asia, and Oceania.[1]

Universal health coverage (UHC) has been policy goal supported by the World Health Organization (WHO),[10] the World Bank,[8] the United Nations (UN),[11] and many governments in LMIC,[12,13] emphasizing propoor progressive universalism, ensuring that coverage includes poor and vulnerable populations.[14] The development of the strategy and pathway to progressive universalism in LMIC is beyond the scope of this article, but, irrespective of the mechanisms by which individual countries move toward UHC, the *Lancet* has recommended a basic level of surgical and anesthesia care to be included as part of the initial coverage package within a country's UHC expansion pathway. The initial coverage packages are designed to provide the most cost-effective interventions and those that are associated with the highest levels of impoverishment in the absence of financial risk protection.[1] Other factors, such as the country's specific context, values, political environment, and resources, should be considered when devising a customized coverage package for each region for which the *Lancet* put forth factors that should be considered when devising surgical and anesthesia care packages within a given region (**Box 2**).[1]

By applying these criteria to LMIC and with emphasis on targeting people in LMIC through the choice of interventions that will benefit them the most, the *Lancet* has devised a set of core surgical procedures, packages, and platforms designed to act as a springboard in the development of these packages in other regions around the globe (**Box 3**).[1] This core package can be tailored further to patients who require oral and maxillofacial surgical care. The basic trauma surgery package within emergency procedures includes open and closed fracture repair, which should include oral and maxillofacial trauma including not only fractures of the craniofacial skeleton (eg, maxilla, mandible, zygomaticomaxillary complex) but soft tissue injuries requiring wound care (eg, laceration repair, skin grafts, local flaps) and debridement. The basic emergency general surgical package includes incision and drainage of soft tissue infections, which should include superficial and deep space head and neck infections of cutaneous and/or odontogenic origin requiring surgical drainage with antibiotic therapy. The general surgical package within planned care packages includes the resection of early-stage oral cavity tumors, whereas the specialist surgical package includes orthognathic surgery, and cleft palate and lip repair. Given the scope of practice of OMS, it should be imperative that dentoalveolar

and an estimated 150 million people face financial catastrophe every year from these OOP costs of medical care.[8,9] Of these 150 million individuals, an estimated 32.8 million cases of catastrophic expenditure occur directly from accessing surgical care,[1] which can lead to decreased life expectancy and economic output. This number represents approximately 22% of the 150 million individuals who endure catastrophic expenditure from accessing all types of health care,[9] which is similar to the proportion of global disease burden that is surgical.[2,4] More alarmingly, between 2015 and 2030, surgical conditions will be responsible for a cumulative loss to the global economy of $20.7 trillion of projected economic output, with neoplasms and injuries requiring surgical care having the greatest effect on economic output.[1] More than half of all of these losses between 2015 and 2030 will occur in LMIC ($12.3

Box 2
Multicriteria decision analysis for funding surgical procedures, packages, and platforms within progressive universalism schemes

Thought should be given to the following factors, using country-specific data and contexts:

- Size of the population affected by the disease
- Severity of the disease, including chance of death or permanent disability if untreated, and including level of impairment
- Effectiveness of the surgical intervention, including chance of cure with the intervention and ability to be done successfully within the skill and resource level of the country
- Economic effect of the condition on the household, including catastrophic expenditure and effect on productivity
- Welfare effect of the condition on the household, including effects on primary caregiver and on schooling and welfare of dependents
- Equity and social implications and the extent to which it is a propoor policy
- Cost-effectiveness of the particular procedure and the platform needed for delivery
- Budget implications of coverage, including necessary expenditure to provide the intervention to all those who need it

From Meara JG, Leather AJM, Hagander L, et al. Global Surgery 2030: evidence and solutions for achieving health, welfare, and economic development. Lancet 2015;386:602; with permission.

Box 3
Core packages for surgical and anesthesia care

The packages listed here would be appropriate to provide within the initial coverage and benefits package under universal health coverage, with examples of procedures each package might cover. Individual countries should perform their own decision analyses to tailor the procedures, packages, and platforms according to their individual needs.

Common conditions: emergency procedures

Basic trauma surgery package

- Open and closed fracture repair, chest tube placement, amputation, trauma laparotomy, burr hole, wound care, debridement

Basic emergency obstetric surgical package

- Caesarean section, hysterectomy, salpingectomy, dilatation and curettage

Basic emergency general surgical package

- Laparotomy, appendectomy, hernia repair with or without bowel resection, incision and drainage of soft tissue infections

Common conditions: planned care packages

General surgical package

- Hernia repair (nonobstructed or incarcerated), hydrocelectomy, cholecystectomy, ureteric or kidney stone removal, prostatectomy, thyroidectomy (goitre-endemic regions), excision biopsy, lumpectomy or mastectomy, resection of early-stage oral cavity tumors, bowel resection

Obstetric and gynecological package

- Treatment of cervical precancerous lesions, hysterectomy for invasive cervical cancer

Specialist surgical package

- Cataract repair, trachoma surgery (where endemic), cleft palate and lip repair, clubfoot correction, surgical repair of congenital heart anomalies, obstetric fistula repair

Palliative surgical care package

- Mastectomy, diversion colostomy; palliative surgical care packages should be delivered alongside access to appropriate palliative analgesics, including opioids

From Meara JG, Leather AJM, Hagander L, et al. Global Surgery 2030: evidence and solutions for achieving health, welfare, and economic development. Lancet 2015;386:602; with permission.

surgery and trauma are included in the context of a planned general surgical package because they are considered to be so-called bread-and-butter procedures of OMS.

Surgical management of oral and maxillofacial disorders requiring complex reconstruction, TMJ dysfunction, and complex craniofacial anomalies should be considered outside the scope of the core package of oral and maxillofacial and anesthesia care under the UHC for LMIC given that these procedures often require multidisciplinary care with specialized instruments and hospital units and are usually considered to be low volume and/or high risk.

CAPACITY BUILDING IN GLOBAL ORAL AND MAXILLOFACIAL SURGERY
Global Surgical Workforce

The WHO published the World Health Report in 2006, identifying a threshold of 228 skilled health professionals per 100,000 population below which countries were unable to reach essential health targets and were deemed to be in a health workforce crisis; as of 2013, 83 countries are still below this threshold.[15,16]

Specialty-specific statistics were obtained by the Lancet Commission and WHO to obtain information on the national and international numbers of specialist surgeons, anesthetists, and obstetricians.[17] The WHO Emergency and Essential Surgical Care (EESC) Programme, which was established to take the lead in efforts to reduce the global burden of surgery-related diseases, has developed the Tool for Situational Analysis to Assess Emergency and Essential Surgical Care and, to date, have collected data from more than 1500 facilities from 62 countries to contribute to the Global Database on EESC.[18] The data from the Lancet Commission and WHO EESC show that only 12% of the specialist surgical workforce practice in Africa and southeast Asia, where one-third of the world's population lives (**Fig. 2**).[17,18] This maldistribution of the specialist surgical workforce, measured by the density of specialist surgeons, anesthetists, and obstetricians per 100,000 population, correlates with specific health outcomes. For example, countries with increased densities of providers per 100,000 population have improved maternal survival, with particularly steep improvements in maternal survival from 0 to roughly 20 specialist providers per 100,000 population. Beyond densities of 40 per 100,000 population, gains are still present, but the gradient of the curve reaches a plateau (**Fig. 3**).[1,19] Based on the UN World Population Prospects to 2030, an estimated 2.28 million specialist surgical, anesthetic, and obstetric providers are needed worldwide to reach the specialist surgical workforce density of 40 per 100,000 population by the year 2030, requiring the surgical workforce to double, at a minimum, in just 15 years.[20] However, for many LMIC, upscaling the specialist surgical workforce to 40 per 100,000 by the year 2030 may not be necessary, and may not be possible. For this reason, the *Lancet* recommends that all countries scale up their surgical workforce to 20 providers per 100,000 population by 2030 as an interim goal, which translates to an additional 1.27 million providers that need to be trained. At present, there are no available data assessing the required workforce density for oral and maxillofacial surgeons; however, the WHO EESC Programme database of needs assessment for surgical and anesthesia services can be tailored to OMS to develop similar databases and global OMS provider density maps to identify regions with greatest need.

Global Surgical Workforce Deficit

Deficits in the global specialist surgical workforce represent multifactorial challenges, mainly in health and education, including infrastructure deficits and financial constraints, leading to a substantial mismatch in workforce supply and demand.[1] Specific factors that contribute to this deficit include an absence of student and trainee exposure to surgery and anesthesia caused by an absence of surgical educators and mentors, facilities, and equipment, which is exacerbated by the presence of greater opportunities for training, career advancement, professional development, and remuneration within the private sector and outside their country of origin in higher-income settings.[21–23] Countries facing substantial workforce shortages are typically caught in a perpetual cycle such that the worsening deficit of the surgical workforce leads to heavier workloads for those who remain, resulting in difficulty achieving quality care and possibly increase the deficit and likelihood for the remaining providers seeking alternative employment opportunities.[1] In turn, students and trainees in that region are likely to be negatively affected by the scarcity of available surgical workforce who have the time and capacity to mentor and educate the next generation of providers, which further reduces the likelihood that students and trainees will enter the surgical workforce or stay in their home countries.[24]

Global Surgical and Oral and Maxillofacial Surgery Workforce Education and Training

At present, there is no comprehensive report on global surgical or oral and maxillofacial surgical workforce training; however, studies have shown that certain similarities of education and training exist across the globe.[1] Most dental and medical schools and training programs are centered in densely populated areas with few located in rural communities where disease types and patient needs might vary and unmet need for care is usually much higher than in urban areas.[1,25]

In an effort to overcome this tremendous gap in the specialist surgical workforce and to quickly and inexpensively expand access to care, many LMIC have engaged in a practice where general practitioners (GPs) and associate clinicians are relied on for surgical and anesthesia care, also known as task shifting and task sharing.[26–28] The Lancet Commission makes a distinction between the 2 terms and emphasizes the shared responsibility of task sharing in which the nonspecialist provider (an associate clinician or GP) ideally has access to consult the specialist surgeon or

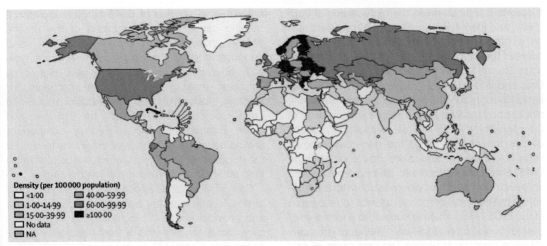

Fig. 2. Global distribution of surgeons, anesthesiologists, and obstetricians per 100,000 population. (*From* Holmer H, Lantz A, Kunjumen T. Global distribution of surgeons, anaesthesiologists, and obstetricians. Lancet Glob Health 2015;3:S10; with permission.)

anesthetist during complicated or unusual procedures.[1]

Task sharing in OMS can be achieved by delegating first-level OMS care to general dentists and/or general surgeons to help close the gap in the OMS workforce, delegating less complex procedures such as dental infections, dentoalveolar surgery, and dental trauma to dentists, and delegating more complex procedures such as deep space cutaneous or odontogenic infections, maxillofacial trauma, and head/neck disorders and reconstruction to general surgeons. The availability of trained oral and maxillofacial surgeons for consultation by dentists and general surgeons for complicated and unusual procedures is crucial to

the safe and effective delivery of standardized care to patients by non–OMS-trained professionals.

The education and training process of OMS varies by country and region across the globe, which may include a dental or medical degree, or both, followed by residency training and options for postresidency fellowship training. Further, management of malignant head and neck tumors is often considered an expanded scope of traditional OMS training in the United States, whereas oral and maxillofacial surgeons are the primary head and neck oncologic surgeons in other parts of the globe. Therefore, global standardization of education training of oral and maxillofacial

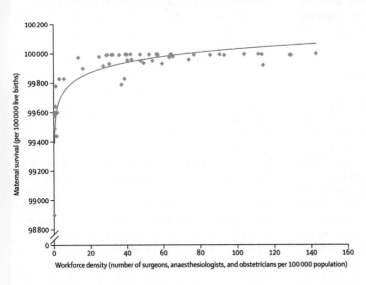

Fig. 3. Specialist surgical workforce density and maternal survival. (*From* Meara JG, Leather AJM, Hagander L, et al. Global Surgery 2030: evidence and solutions for achieving health, welfare, and economic development. Lancet 2015;386:588; with permission.)

surgeons is difficult given the high degree of variability, and identifying qualified OMS professionals on a global standard can be challenging. To address this high degree of variability, the International Board for the Certification of Specialists in Oral and Maxillofacial Surgery (IBCSOMS) was established in 2015 to improve the welfare of the global community by improving the standards of the specialty of OMS.[29] This certification process verifies the attainment of the necessary knowledge, experience, and skills for specialists in OMS, and a commitment to lifelong learning and contemporary practice, where successful completion of the certification process leads to fellowship of the IBCSOMS, which is subject to a formal process of periodic reevaluation.[30] Although this certification process improves the standards of oral and maxillofacial surgical care on a global scale, mandating additional certification in order to practice OMS may lead to additional shortages of these specialized surgeons in many LMIC.

Capacity Building in the Global Oral and Maxillofacial Surgery Workforce

Efforts to scale up the global OMS workforce to provide quality care must not only be undertaken by the LMIC in need but should be considered a global effort with assistance from high-income countries. Standards of care can be established by accreditation of LMIC medical and dental schools in addition to postgraduate training programs because the quality of trainees who graduate from nonaccredited programs may be compromised.[1] LMIC should also plan the entering and exiting of OMS professionals in the workforce with careful consideration along the entire dental and/or medical education, postgraduate training, and workforce pipeline to ensure that the density, distribution, and undertaking of the surgical workforce is aligned with population needs.

Academic dental and medical institutions and training programs in high-income countries also have an important role in the scale-up of the global OMS workforce. Although humanitarian surgical missions are not considered requirements based on the standards of the Council of Dental Accreditation (CODA) for OMS training in the United Sates, there is a growing interest and emphasis on the value of OMS trainees on humanitarian missions.[31] These missions provide an opportunity for bidirectional learning to take place, where the educational benefit does not only apply to the visiting OMS trainee but is also an opportunity for trainees in the host country to learn from the OMS workforce from high-income countries. The

breadth and volume of OMS surgical workforce training can include the support of the private sector, nonprofit organizations (NPOs) and nongovernmental organizations, which are typically adequately resourced and have high case volumes, making them rich environments for learning,[1] as seen in such organizations as Smile Train, Operation Smile, Healing the Children, and Smile Bangladesh, and a training component should be hardwired into their programs to ensure the durability of their effect, which will be sustained long after the organization has left the region.[1]

Smile Train has developed several training programs to enhance the training of local surgeons and providers in LMIC, including the Virtual Surgery Simulator, which is a freely available, Web-accessible surgical simulator providing instruction for cleft lip and palate surgical repair, and hands-on quality-improvement training and surgical training exchange programs, which are one-on-one training programs, and small group workshops designed to improve surgical outcomes across partner networks.[32]

In conjunction with the Bangladeshi Association of Oral and Maxillofacial Surgeons, Smile Bangladesh has established an orthognathic surgery training program in Bangladesh where US oral and maxillofacial surgeons collaborate with local Bangladeshi oral and maxillofacial surgeons and trainees in Dhaka-based medical and dental teaching institutions to implement an orthognathic surgery curriculum. This biannual program spanning 7 to 10 days includes lectures, cadaver dissections, model surgery, virtual surgical planning, and live surgery, with each program focusing on various topics and surgical techniques to provide a comprehensive orthognathic surgery training program for local OMS surgeons and trainees.

However, short-term, humanitarian missions sponsored by high-income countries are often not adequate in the training of surgical specialists in LMIC. To address the health disparities associated with inadequate access to surgical care in LMIC through a long-term program, the Paul Farmer Global Surgery Fellowship was created in an effort to not only bring to light the growing health, surgical and anesthesia, and economic disparities in LMIC but to train leaders who will focus on developing the skill set necessary to promote the role of surgical care, education, and research pertinent to global surgery, anesthesia, and obstetrics/gynecologic care in health systems, and strengthening UHC.[33] The program, which is 12 to 24 months in duration, allows surgical fellows to operate independently in collaboration with their in-country partners to provide surgical care in resource-poor international sites and gain firsthand experience in surgical program development, public health, human rights, and education of local providers.[33]

For oral and maxillofacial surgeons, IAOMS offers several 12-month surgical fellowships for senior trainees and recent graduates from OMS programs around the globe, focusing on head/neck oncology and microvascular reconstruction, and cleft lip/palate and craniofacial surgery.[34] The *American College of Surgeons Bulletin* is also a valuable resource for surgeons, including oral and maxillofacial surgeons, interested in capacity building to seek and create OMS fellowships and forming partnerships with academic institutions, NPOs, and public and private foundations to help sustain these projects.[35]

These programs provide OMS trainees from LMIC an opportunity to further develop their training in OMS subspecialties with which they can return to their home countries to not only provide specialized OMS care to patients but, more importantly, train the next generation of oral and maxillofacial surgeons.

Financial resources and funding for specialist surgical education and training, including the funding of humanitarian missions and surgical fellowships, often act as a barrier for individuals who wish to enter the global specialist surgical workforce. In an effort to minimize or offset these costs, partnerships between high-income countries and LMIC where financial, technical, and specialist support is provided to enhance surgical training have proved to be beneficial to trainees from LMIC, as shown by the partnership established between the Uganda Society of Anaesthesia and the Association of Anaesthetists of Great Britain to financially and educationally support postgraduate anesthesia training in Uganda.[1,21] These partnerships should also be considered for the education and training in OMS originating from LMIC. For OMS trainees and surgeons, financial scholarship programs are available through professional OMS organizations, such as the American Association of Oral and Maxillofacial Surgeons (AAOMS) and the Oral and Maxillofacial Surgery Foundation (OMSF), which provide funding for humanitarian missions and fellowships.[36,37]

Research in Global Surgery and Global Oral and Maxillofacial Surgery

There is a paucity of data in global surgery research with a focus on practices and capacity because, historically, global health research efforts have not focused on diseases with the highest burden or on regions with the greatest clinical need.[1,38–40] This problem is exacerbated by clinicians who are trained to do research being concentrated in higher-income regions, with only an estimated 13% of the world's scientists located in Africa, Latin America, and the Middle East.[41] This finding shows that the highest volume of surgical research is not done in, or by, the countries with the greatest clinical need; rather, surgical research output correlates with the total gross domestic product.[1]

Global surgery research in the past has focused largely on bringing to light the importance of surgery, the absence of infrastructure, and the cost-effectiveness of surgical intervention; however, focus on the development of solutions to these challenges is crucial.[1] The development of these solutions will only be possible with the collaboration between local and global partners, ministries of health, academic institutions, funding partners, and global health institutions.[1]

The Lancet Commission has set forth a research agenda based on data and knowledge gaps identified during the commission process, to help maximize the global surgery research effort, which are as follows:[1]

1. The prevalence of surgical conditions affecting the world population to identify regions of greatest need for allocation of resources should be identified, because data pertaining to the burden of surgical conditions are scarce.
2. Identifying the determinants (social, occupational, environmental, genetic, geographic, and demographic) of surgical disease and barriers to care will help tailor appropriate strategies to improve access, delivery, and prevention.
3. LMIC-specific research is needed, investigating how financing of surgical care can be used to improve efficiency and performance and achieve economies of scope and scale with optimum returns on investment.
4. Additional research to define feasible and effective strategies and best-practice protocols for surgical and anesthesia care delivery in LMIC is crucial because much of the research into safety in surgery is based on high-resource settings, and the increasing focus on LMIC has been valuable but mainly limited to pulse oximetry and safety checklists.
5. Research on methods for establishing reliable supply chains for surgical equipment, supplies, and drugs; safe waste disposal; and diagnostics, including pathology, laboratory, and imaging capabilities, should be included to improve care delivery in LMIC.

This agenda should be tailored to answer research questions for capacity building in global

OMS and in the context of available resources and needs for a given region and for LMIC.

Future Directions of Global Oral and Maxillofacial Surgery

Surgery on a global scale has long been overlooked as a necessity in health care for the world's poorest populations, where 9 out of 10 people across the globe do not have access to basic surgical care. Global oral and maxillofacial surgical care is included in the global burden of surgical disease, and increased awareness of the need for global OMS is a necessity. The initiation, support, and funding of research on the global burden of oral and maxillofacial surgical conditions to develop a global OMS capacity-building strategy is imperative. Reaching this goal by the year 2030 will require the collaboration and partnerships of public and private sectors, academic institutions, and professional dental and medical associations with industry and philanthropy funding to develop capacity building and needs and outcomes assessments to provide universal oral and maxillofacial surgical care for all.

DISCLOSURE

The authors have nothing to disclose.

REFERENCES

1. Meara JG, Leather AJM, Hagander L, et al. Global Surgery 2030: evidence and solutions for achieving health, welfare, and economic development. Lancet 2015;386:569–624.
2. Shrime MG, Bickler WS, Alkire BC, et al. Global burden of surgical disease: an estimation from the provider perspective. Lancet Glob Health 2015;3: S8–9.
3. Lozano R, Naghavi M, Foreman K, et al. Global and regional mortality from 235 causes of death for 20 age groups in 1990 and 2010: a systematic analysis for the Global Burden of Disease Study 2010. Lancet 2012;380:2095–128.
4. Bickler SW, Weiser TG, Kassebaum N, et al. Global burden of surgical conditions. In: Debas HT, Donkor P, Gawande A, et al, editors. Disease control priorities, 3rd edition, vol 1. Essential surgery. Washington, DC: World Bank; 2015. p. 9–40.
5. Byass P. The imperfect world of global health estimates. PLoS Med 2010;7:e1001006.
6. Kim JY, Farmer P, Porter ME. Redefining global health-care delivery. Lancet 2013;382:1060–9.
7. Mendis S, Fukino K, Cameron A, et al. The availability and affordability of selected essential medicines for chronic diseases in six low- and middle-income countries. Bull World Health Organ 2007;85:279–88.
8. Kutzin J. Towards universal health care coverage: a goal-oriented framework for policy analysis. Washington, DC: World Bank; 2000.
9. Xu K, Evans DB, Kawabata K, et al. Household catastrophic health expenditure: a multicountry analysis. Lancet 2003;362:111–7.
10. WHO. Health systems financing: the path to universal coverage. Geneva (Switzerland): World Health Organization; 2010.
11. Vega J. Universal health coverage: the post-2015 development agenda. Lancet 2013;381:179–80.
12. Makaka A, Breen S, Binagwaho A. Universal health coverage in Rwanda: a report of innovations to increase enrolment in community-based health insurance. Lancet 2012;380:S7.
13. Lagomarsino G, Garabrant A, Adyas A, et al. Moving towards universal health coverage: health insurance reforms in nine developing countries in Africa and Asia. Lancet 2012;380:933–43.
14. Jamison DT, Summers LH, Alleyne G, et al. Global health2035: a world converging within a generation. Lancet 2013;382:1898–955.
15. WHO. The world health report 2006: working together for health. Geneva (Switzerland): World Health Organization; 2006. Available at: http://www.who.int/whr/2006/whr06_en.pdf. Accessed December 21, 2019.
16. Campbell J, Dussault G, Buchan J, et al. A universal truth: No health without a workforce. Third global Forum on human resources for health. Recife (Brazil): World Health Organization; 2013. Available at: https://www.who.int/workforcealliance/knowledge/resources/GHWA_AUniversalTruthReport.pdf. Accessed December 21, 2019.
17. Holmer H, Lantz A, Kunjumen T, et al. Global distribution of surgeons, anaesthesiologists, and obstetricians. Lancet Glob Health 2015;3:S9–11.
18. World Health Organization. Essential and emergency surgical care. Available at: https://www.who.int/surgery/en/. Accessed February 2, 2020.
19. Holmer H, Shrime M, Riesel JN, et al. Towards closing the gap of the global surgeon, anaesthesiologist and obstetrician workforce: thresholds and projections towards 2030. Lancet 2015;385(Global Surgery special issue):S40.
20. UN World Population Prospects. The 2012 revision. Available at: https://www.un.org/en/development/desa/publications/world-population-prospects-the-2012-revision.html. Accessed December 21, 2019.
21. Bajunirwe F, Twesigye L, Zhang M, et al. Influence of the US President's Emergency Plan for AIDS Relief (PEPfAR) on career choices and emigration of health-profession graduates from a Ugandan medical school: a cross-sectional study. BMJ Open 2013;3:e002875.
22. Abioye IA, Ibrahim NA, Odesanya MO, et al. The future of trauma care in a developing country:

interest of medical students and interns in surgery and surgical specialties. Int J Surg 2012;10:209–12.

23. Kahn D, Pillay S, Veller MG, et al. General surgery in crisis—comparatively low levels of remuneration. S Afr J Surg 2006;44:96, 98–99,102.

24. Burch VC, McKinley D, van Wyk J, et al. Career intentions of medical students trained in six sub-Saharan African countries. Educ Health (Abingdon) 2011;24:614.

25. Atiyeh BS, Gunn SWA, Hayek SN. Provision of essential surgery in remote and rural areas of developed as well as low and middle income countries. Int J Surg 2010;8:581–5.

26. Mkandawire N, Ngulube C, Lavy C. Orthopaedic clinical officer program in Malawi: a model for providing orthopaedic care. Clin Orthop Relat Res 2008;466:2385–91.

27. Chilopora G, Pereira C, Kamwendo F, et al. Postoperative outcome of caesarean sections and other major emergency obstetric surgery by clinical officers and medical officers in Malawi. Hum Resour Health 2007;5:17.

28. Pereira C, Cumbi A, Malalane R, et al. Meeting the need for emergency obstetric care in Mozambique: work performance and histories of medical doctors and assistant medical officers trained for surgery. BJOG 2007;114:1530–3.

29. IBCSOMS History. Available at: https://www.ibcsoms.org/WebPages/History.aspx. Accessed January 11, 2020.

30. International Board of the Certification of Specialists in Oral and Maxillofacial Surgery. 2019 Certification Handbook. Available at: https://www.ibcsoms.org/Admin/AdminAttachments/2019CandidateHandbook.pdf. Accessed January 11, 2020.

31. Aziz SR, Ziccardi VB, Chuang SK. Survey of residents who have participated in humanitarian medical missions. J Oral Maxillofac Surg 2012;70:e147–57.

32. Smile train training programs. Available at: https://www.smiletrain.org/cleft-resources/training-programs. Accessed January 25, 2020.

33. Paul Farmer Global Surgery Research Fellowship. Available at: https://www.pgssc.org/paul-farmer-global-surgery-fellowship. Accessed January 25, 2020.

34. IAOMS Foundation Programs. Available at: https://www.iaoms.org/iaoms-foundation/programs. Accessed January 25, 2020.

35. American College of Surgeons. Above and beyond: a primer for young surgeons interested in global surgery. Available at: https://bulletin.facs.org/2017/02/above-and-beyond-a-primer-for-young-surgeons-interested-in-global-surgery. Accessed February 2, 2020.

36. AAOMS Global Outreach Program. Available at: https://www.aaoms.org/member-center/global-outreach-program. Accessed January 11, 2020.

37. OMSF Global Initiative for Volunteerism and Education (GIVE). Available at: https://omsfoundation.org/research-education/funding/give. Accessed January 11, 2020.

38. Elobu AE, Kintu A, Galukande M, et al. Evaluating international global health collaborations: perspectives from surgery and anesthesia trainees in Uganda. Surgery 2014;155:585–92.

39. Røttingen JA, Regmi S, Eide M, et al. Mapping of available health research and development data: what's there, what's missing, and what role is there for a global observatory? Lancet 2013;382:1286–307.

40. Moran M, Guzman J, Chapman N, et al. Neglected disease research and development: the public divide. Australia: G-Finder. 2013. Available at: http://www.policycures.org/downloads/GF_report13_all_web.pdf. Accessed January 11, 2020.

41. Nordberg E, Holmberg S, Kiugu S. Output of major surgery in developing countries. Towards a quantitative evaluation and planning tool. Trop Geogr Med 1995;47:206–11.

Global Burden of Head and Neck Cancer

Quazi Billur Rahman, MD, PGD, PhD[a], Oreste Iocca, DDS, MD[b], Kenneth Kufta, DMD, MD[c], Rabie M. Shanti, DMD, MD[c],*

KEYWORDS

- Head and neck cancer • Global burden of cancer • Tobacco • Human papilloma virus • Oral cancer
- Oropharyngeal cancer

KEY POINTS

- Cancer is the leading cause of death in countries with developed economies.
- Tobacco use is responsible for the majority of the global burden of head and neck cancer.
- Tobacco use is increasing in developing economies, contributing the increasing burden of head and neck cancer, especially oral cancer.
- Human papilloma virus is responsible for the dramatic increase in the incidence of oropharyngeal cancer in Western countries.

INTRODUCTION

Cancer refers to a group of diseases characterized by uncontrolled or unchecked division of cells with the potential for these cells to metastasize. Cancer imparts a significant degree of emotional stress, psychological trauma, physical discomfort, and financial hardship on society; it is a major source of morbidity and mortality worldwide among all age groups. Today, cancer is the leading cause of death in countries with developed economies and is the second leading cause of death in countries with developing economies.[1] Furthermore, countries with developed economies have an incidence of cancer that is nearly twice as high as that of economically developing countries.[1] A myriad of factors is contributing to the increasing global burden of cancer, all of which are interconnected to increases in human development. These variables include an aging population, population growth,

lifestyle changes, economic variables, and societal changes.[2] For instance, as economies transition and become more economically prosperous, the incidence of cancer increases, and more specifically these increases are in cancers (eg, breast, prostate, colorectal) that are more common in high-income countries.[3] Furthermore, as countries continue to develop economically, the incidence of certain infection-based cancers (eg, Kaposi sarcoma and cervical and liver cancers) decrease over time.[3]

It is estimated that the burden of cancer will continue to increase, with global estimates of 22 million new cancer cases (compared with an estimated 14 million cases in 2012) and 13 million cancer-related deaths occurring annually by 2030.[2–4] Therefore, in this article we review the emerging trends in various subsites of head and neck cancer on a global scale. This information is valuable to oral and maxillofacial surgeons, because we are global practitioners and leaders

[a] Department of Oral and Maxillofacial Surgery, Bangabandhu Sheikh Mujib Medical University (BSMMU), Room – 303, Block A, Shahbag, Dhaka 1000, Bangladesh; [b] Department of Otolaryngology—Head and Neck Surgery, Humanitas Clinical and Research Center, IRCCS, via Manzoni 56, 20089 Rozzano (MI), Italy; [c] Department of Oral and Maxillofacial Surgery and Pharmacology, School of Dental Medicine, University of Pennsylvania, Perelman Center for Advanced Medicine, 3400 Civic Center Blvd, 4th Floor South Pavilion, Philadelphia, PA, 19104, USA
* Corresponding author.
E-mail address: Rabie.Shanti@pennmedicine.upenn.edu

Oral Maxillofacial Surg Clin N Am 32 (2020) 367–375
https://doi.org/10.1016/j.coms.2020.04.002
1042-3699/20/© 2020 Elsevier Inc. All rights reserved.

in the diagnosis and management of cancers of the head and neck, and it is imperative that we stay abreast of the changing global health care landscape for us to continue to contribute to and lead the care of patients suffering from head and neck cancer.

ORAL CAVITY AND OROPHARYNGEAL CANCERS

Oral cavity and oropharyngeal cancers combined make up the sixth most common cancer subsite in the world. In 2012 it was estimated that 443,000 new cases of oral and oropharyngeal cancer were diagnosed, and 241,450 deaths were attributed to cancers of the oral cavity and oropharynx.[4,5] By 2018, the incidence increased to 710,000 and the number of deaths attributed to the oral cavity and oropharyngeal cancers was 350,000.[5,6] Although these disease burden rates are global figures, the incidence of oral cancer in some parts of the world is decreasing largely owing to decreases in tobacco use.[7,8] However, secondary to human papilloma virus (HPV) infection several countries (ie, the United States, Canada, Australia, Sweden, Netherlands, Denmark, and the UJ) over the past 2 decades have experienced an increase in the incidence of oropharyngeal cancer, especially in men less than 60 years of age.[7,8] Although most reported cancer statistics combine the oral cavity proper and oropharynx proper in reporting epidemiologic data, from a clinical perspective these 2 subsites are staged differently and guidelines for their management and prognostication are significantly different. Therefore, we discuss them separately from here on.

Oral Cancer

The oral cavity is the most common subsite of head and neck mucosal malignancies. In the Unites States oral cancer makes up approximately 5% of cancers, whereas in India it is the most common form of cancer, accounting for 35% to 40% of all malignancies.[9] This widely varying incidence of oral cancer has been attributed mainly to the use of spices (ie, betel nut) and to a lesser degree untreated syphilis in India and Pakistan in comparison with North American and European countries.[10] Varying social behaviors and customs contributing to oral cancer prevalence have been observed even in countries that are geographically closer to one another. For instance, in Eastern Europe (ie, Slovakia and Slovenia) and France, oral cancer has a much higher incidence than Western European countries owing to greater consumption of tobacco and alcohol. Although alcohol is a known risk factor for oral cancer, with individuals consuming

more than 170 g of whisky daily having a 10-fold greater risk for the development of oral cancer, the primary risk factor for the global burden of oral cancer remains tobacco.[11,12] Although the carcinogenic properties of tobacco are well understood, the delivery of tobacco varies based on local social practices within a country or particular pockets of a country. Today, the most common form of tobacco use is in the form of smoking. Areca nut chewing is also responsible for a significant portion of the global burden of oral cancer. For example, in Taiwan 85% of patients diagnosed with oral cancer have the habit of chewing on Areca nut.[9] Areca nut is a fruit that is considered a psychoactive substance, and its extract is composed of saccharides, fats, polyphenols, various alkaloids, tannins, and crude fiber (**Fig. 1**).[9] The areca nut can be covered with betel leaves or inflorescence to form betel quids for chewing.[9] Betel nuts originated in South East Asia and India, and the chewing of betel nut is practiced throughout parts of Asia and the East Indies.[13] As discussed elsewhere in this article, a betel nut is made up of areca nut and betel leaf, but can also contain other ingredients, such as catechu, slaked lime, and spices or sweeteners (eg, cloves, fennel, cardamom, coconut, and aniseed).[13] The quid is usually placed in the buccal sulcus and is frequently kept in the mouth for several hours for several hours per day, resulting in squamous cell carcinoma of the gingivobuccal sulcus (**Fig. 2**). As the quid is chewed, alkaloids are released from the areca nut and the tobacco, which are said to aid in digestion of foods and to also result in a euphoric state. Often the habit begins in childhood, and the frequency of use increases with age. A multitude of studies have demonstrated that betel nut and the areca nut can induce premalignant and malignant changes of the oral epithelium. For example, a person who chews less than 10 quids per day has a 26.4 greater risk for development of oral cancer, and a person who chews more than 20 quids per day has a 275.6 times greater risk for the development of oral cancer.[14] Moreover, several of the components (ie, catechins, tannins, flavonoids) of these substances can facilitate the cross-linking of collagen fibers, increase collagen levels through activation of the transforming growth factor-beta pathway, and also decrease susceptibility to collagenases, resulting in the development of oral submucosal fibrosis (**Fig. 3**).[9]

The potency of carcinogenesis of betel quid use explains the global burden of oral cancer in specific parts of Asia (ie, India, Pakistan, and Taiwan); however, tobacco smoking remains the major contributor for the vast majority of oral cancer cases worldwide. Other forms of tobacco the are

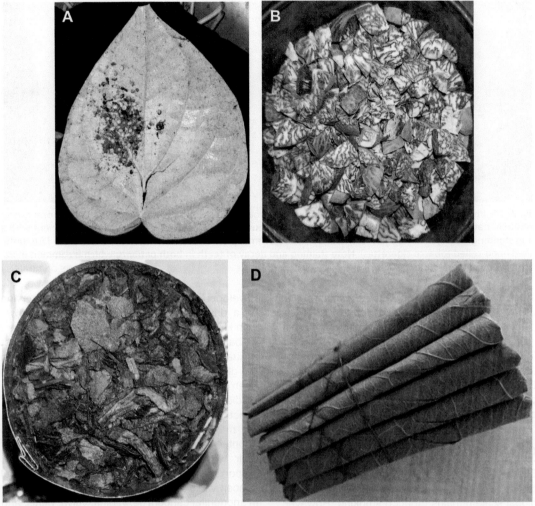

Fig. 1. (*A*) Betel leaf. (*B*) Areca nut. (*C*) Smokeless tobacco (Zarda, chopped tobacco leaves with aromatic ingredients and *Shada*, dried raw chopped tobacco leaves), and (*D*) *Bidi*, a form of unfiltered smoking tobacco that is made of unprocessed tobacco wrapped in leaves.

commonly used in South Asian countries such as Bangladesh, India, Pakistan, and Sri Lanka include *Bidis* and *Gul* (see **Fig. 2**B, **Fig. 4**). Although some Western countries have demonstrated a decrease in the prevalence of tobacco smoking, unfortunately there is an increasing trend in the use of tobacco in certain parts of the world, which is shifting the burden of oral cancer to developing countries. For instance, current World Health Organization (WHO) estimates are that approximately 80% of the world's smokers reside in low-income and middle-income countries.[5]

With these changing trend, what does the global landscape look like today as it relates to the geographic distribution of oral cancer? According to the International Association of Cancer Registries, a component of the WHO via the GLOBO-CAN project, the greatest burden of oral cancer in the world is in South Asian countries, such as India, Pakistan, Bangladesh, and Sri Lanka, where one-third of all cancers are oral cancers.[15,16] Among South Asian countries, Sri Lanka had the highest incidence of oral cancer, followed by Pakistan.[15,17] Furthermore, as result of these changing trends in tobacco consumption, the United States has been experiencing a 1.5% annual percentage decrease in oral cancer incidence, and France has been experiencing a 1% annual percentage decrease.[15,18] Hungary, which is considered an "upper" middle-income country, has experience a 2-fold increase in the incidence of oral cancer.[15,18]

In summary, as oral and maxillofacial surgeons, we are to anticipate a global increase in the incidence of oral cancer, and oral cancer related mortality. To date, one of the most impactful means of

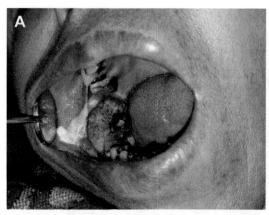
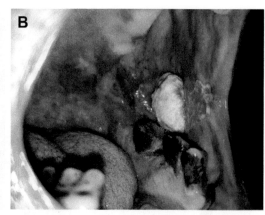

Fig. 2. (A) Invasive squamous cell carcinoma of the gingivobuccal sulcus, which is the most common oral cancer subsite in patients who use smokeless tobacco. (B) Verrucous carcinoma of left buccal mucosa in a patient with a long standing history of betel quid use with a mixture of smokeless tobacco and areca nut, as well as *Bidi* (unfiltered hand-rolled tobacco cigarettes). Note staining and decay of teeth in both patients, which is common in patients who use betel quid.

reducing the incidence of oral cancer has been decrease in tobacco use; therefore, we must continue to work closely with our health care organizations, advocacy groups, and educational platforms to play a part in the decrease of tobacco use. Based on global figures it seems that low- to middle-income countries are the ones that will be impact the most in future with increasing burdens of oral cancer.

Oropharynx Cancer

Similar to oral cancer, the primary risk factor for the development of oropharyngeal cancer on a global scale remains tobacco smoking. However, the epidemiologic landscape of oropharyngeal cancer is rapidly changing with HPV emerging as the key etiologic driver for the majority of newly diagnosed oropharyngeal cancers, specifically in

developed countries.[19] The role of HPV in serving as a driver for cancer formation is well-known, with HPV-associated cancers posing a significant global health burden.[20] HPV is one of the most sexually transmitted infections worldwide, with the global HPV prevalence among women having been estimated to be around 11.7%, based on studies using cervical cytologic findings.[21] HPV infection does not usually illicit symptoms, with the majority of patients resolving their infection spontaneously. Women are more likely to clear their HPV infection than men. Today, HPV is responsible for essentially all cases of cervical cancer, while also serving as a key etiologic factor in anogenital cancers (ie, vagina, vulva, penis, and anus) and oropharyngeal cancer.[22]

With more than 200 HPV types having been identified to date, the majority of the global health burden of HPV-related cancers is attributable to a

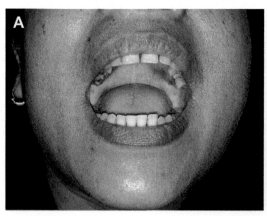
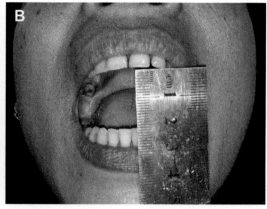

Fig. 3. (A) Clinical photograph of a patient with of submucous fibrosis owing to chewing of areca nut for a duration of 20 years. (B) Trismus, very common sequela of oral submucosal fibrosis.

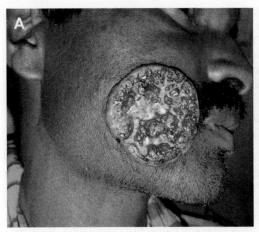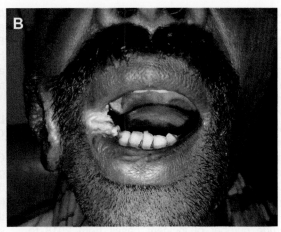

Fig. 4. (A, B) Squamous cell carcinoma of the right buccal mucosal invasion of cheek in a patient who uses *Gul*, which is a powder form of dried raw tobacco that people place along and/or rub against oral tissues (ie, gingiva).

few HPV types.[22] Today, the role of HPV in carcinogenesis is well-established with more than 90% of cases of HPV-associated oropharyngeal cancer being attributed to HPV 16; however, other HPV types have been implicated in cancer, including HPV types 18, 31, 33, 35, 39, 45, 51, 52, 56, 58, and 59.[19,21] HPV types 16 and 18 are also the primary drivers of anogenital and cervical cancer owing to their high carcinogenic capacity.[22] HPV 16 has been detected in 3.2% and HPV 18 in 1.4% of women worldwide.[21,22]

As one would expect, and similar to tobacco consumption, regional distribution differences with regard to HPV prevalence do exist. Sub-Saharan Africa, Latin America, the Caribbean, Eastern Europe, and Southeastern Asian have the highest documented prevalences of HPV infection based on cytologic data in women.[21] The prevalence of HPV infection has added to the global burden of head and neck cancers, with oropharyngeal squamous cell carcinoma increasing. For instance, in the United States, there has been nearly a 50% increase in the numbers of newly diagnosed cases of oropharyngeal squamous cell carcinoma.[23] Furthermore, Danish cancer registries have reported a 5% to 8% annual increase in the incidence of HPV-positive oropharyngeal cancer.[23–25] In Asia, Taiwan and Korea have experienced a 6.9% and 2.4% increase, respectively.[26,27]

The first prophylactic virus-like particle vaccine for HPV was introduced in 2006, with the initial HPV vaccine trials using both a bivalent and quadrivalent HPV vaccine for HPV types 16 and 18 and HPV types 6, 11, 16, and 18, respectively.[28,29] As discussed elsewhere in this article, HPV types 16 and 18 are the most oncogenic HPV types, whereas HPV types 6 and 11 are responsible for

approximately 90% cases of genital warts.[28,30,31] Subsequently in 2014, the nonavalent HPV vaccine was first registered for clinical use, with this vaccine also containing virus-like particles for HPV types 6, 11, 16, and 18 and also for the next 5 most commonly detected HPV types in cervical cancer: HPV types 31, 33, 45, 52, and 58.[28] To date, a myriad of studies have proved the safety and high efficacy of HPV vaccines, with countries that have implemented robust population-based programs showing a substantial decline in HPV infection.[28] For instance, the effectiveness of the quadrivalent HPV vaccine has been demonstrated in decreasing the incidence of genital warts in Italy (men and women), Denmark (men and women), Canada (women only), and Israel (men and women).[28,32–35]

Although the role of HPV as an etiologic factor in oropharyngeal cancer is clear, one must not forget that tobacco smoking still plays a significant role as a risk factor for the development of HPV-negative and HPV-positive oropharyngeal cancers.[36] Therefore, the incidence of HPV-positive oropharyngeal cancer was found to be higher in ever smokers in comparison with never smokers, as well as being higher in current smokers versus former smokers.[36]

NASOPHARYNGEAL CANCER

Squamous cell carcinoma of the nasopharynx is relatively rare when compared with other head and neck subsites. It is classified into 3 major histologic subtypes: keratinizing, nonkeratinizing, and basaloid. The WHO Global Cancer Observatory[17] reports that the overall incidence of new nasopharyngeal cancer cases in 2018 was 129,079, with 72,987 related deaths. It is well-known that the majority of new cases occur in Eastern and South-Eastern Asia with 64,304 (lifetime cumulative risk 0.29%) and 34,681 (lifetime cumulative risk 0.55%) new cases, respectively. In detail, in Southern China its incidence reaches a peak of 20 in 100,000, compared with 0.5 to 1 in 100,000 in Europe and North America. The male-to-female ratio is 2 to 3:1, with slight variations according to the geographic regions examined. In the last 2 decades, a decrease in incidence has been observed in the high incidence areas, with average annual changes of −2% in Chinese males, −3.3% in Chinese females, and overall annual decrease spanning from −1% to −5% worldwide.[37] Nevertheless, the estimated crude number of incident cases from 2018 to 2040, for both sexes and all ages, is predicted to increase, likely owing to the expansion of the population worldwide. The global cancer observatory predicts 158,558 new nasopharynx cancer cases and 93,338 related deaths in 2030.[17]

Given the peculiar epidemiologic characteristics of nasopharynx carcinoma, investigators have been focused on particular risk factors that may be linked to this pathologic entity. It is now clear that Epstein-Barr virus (EBV), acting in synergy with the other risk factors like tobacco, salted food, and alcohol, plays a major role in tumorigenesis.[38] It is possible that specific HLA haplotypes play a role in the etiology of nasopharyngeal cancer, and this may explain why particular populations are more susceptible than others to the occurrence of the disease.[39] It is worth noting that recent research[40] suggests an increase in EBV-related incidence in the United States, in particular, the nonkeratinizing subtype. It has been estimated that the average age at diagnosis in the United States is 55 years, although in patients of African American descent a bimodal distribution was noted, with a greater proportion of younger patients diagnosed with nasopharyngeal cancer compared with their white counterparts. This finding is likely due to the established higher rate of EBV infection among African Americans.

In general, worldwide mortality has shown favorable trends in the last decades and the 5-year prevalence in 2018 has been estimated to be 362,219. This finding is also due to a better understanding of the optimal treatment modalities based on concurrent chemoradiotherapy and, in selected cases, induction chemotherapy.[41] It is possible that a change in lifestyle, dietary habits, and improved diagnostic accuracy, especially in high incidence areas, has contributed to these favorable trends. Further decreases of the global burden of this pathologic entity depends on the decrease of smoking habits, alcohol consumption, and preserved food intake. Finally, a future understanding of the molecular role of EBV in the interaction with these risk factors will help in developing mass screening programs and effective preventive measures in high-risk areas of the world.

LARYNGEAL AND HYPOPHARYNGEAL CANCERS

Cancers of the larynx and hypopharynx are often grouped together for anatomic reasons. Although they likely share common etiologic factors (alcohol, tobacco, and areca nut chewing being the predominant ones), these are 2 distinct entities with a different mode of presentation, treatment approaches, and prognosis.

Hypopharynx cancer is uncommon and, given to its silent growth in the initial stages, it is often discovered late in the course of the disease,[42] which leads to a poor prognosis. The WHO Global Cancer Observatory[17] reports 80,608 new cases worldwide in 2018; the highest incidence is in South-Central Asia with 36,835 cases and a lifetime cumulative risk of being affected of 0.25%, compared with 3125 new cases in North America (lifetime cumulative risk 0.06%), 7079 in Central and Eastern Europe (lifetime cumulative risk 0.12%), and 6249 in Western Europe (lifetime cumulative risk 0.22%). The male-to-female ratio incidence is 5:1 worldwide. A recent report[43] collected the data coming from national cancer registries of various countries from 1978 up to 2011. It was outlined that, in general, the number of new cases was stable across the decades, with limited geographic variations. It was noted that there is a lower incidence of hypopharyngeal cancer in the Southern parts of the world.

It is likely that, with the improvements in therapeutic options, combining surgery and chemoradiotherapy,[44] the prevalence of this cancer will increase, the global cancer observatory currently estimates its 5-year prevalence to be 119,130 worldwide.

Larynx cancer is more common; its incidence has been estimated to be 177,422 in 2018.[17] The number of new cases in North America was of 16,352 (lifetime cumulative risk of 0.32%), in South Central Asia of 42,439 (lifetime cumulative risk of 0.30%), and in Eastern Asia of 34,409 (lifetime cumulative risk of 0.16%). Eastern and Central Europe recorded 18,028 new cases in 2018, which is the highest lifetime cumulative risk of all regions with 0.46%; this is likely due to a higher prevalence of smokers and/or heavy drinkers in these areas. The male-to-female ratio is around 6:1 globally.

Recent evidence suggests that there is a wide disparity in worldwide incidence, treatment, and survival for larynx cancer between urban and rural areas.[45] This is also true in developed countries like the United States, in which the authors found out that the age-adjusted incidence rates of larynx cancer in large urban, urban nonmetropolitan, and rural areas were respectively 2.8, 3.8, and 4.5 per 100,000. In contrast, survival after diagnosis in different areas of the United States was comparable.

The treatment options for larynx cancer have improved significantly over the past 3 decades, with the development of partial laryngectomies techniques, larynx preservation chemoradiotherapy treatment options,[46] and better management of recurrent disease.[47] Cancer survival aside, larynx survivorship poses the unique challenge of maintaining an acceptable quality of life given the importance of this organ for phonation and respiration. The estimated 5-year worldwide prevalence[17] of 488,900 patients makes it evident that the larynx cancer burden is a challenge for the multidisciplinary team involved in its management. This finding is true in developed and underdeveloped countries alike.

SINONASAL CANCER

Sinonasal cancers are malignancies of the nasal cavity as well as accessory sinus cavity of the face. Internationally, sinonasal cancers constitute about 0.2% of all cancers.[48] Studies have found that the majority of these cancers affect the nasal cavity (44%–46%) and maxillary sinus (29%–36%), with less than 10% affecting frontal, ethmoid, and sphenoid sinuses.[49] Based on WHO statistics taken from the GLOBOCAN dataset for 9 countries, the overall incidence was found to be 5 to 9 per million for males and 2 to 5 per million for females, with most tumors occurs in individuals greater than 65 years of age.[48] The incidence was shown to be 0.556 to 0.83 cases per 100,000 people per year in the United States.[49,50] There is a propensity for these tumors to affect males, with a 2:1 male:female incidence ratio.[49] This incidence in the United States has remained stable from 1973 to 2006, without a significant change in the overall prognosis (5-year survival rate of about 55%).[49] Regarding the global burden of sinonasal cancers, there has been a general decrease in the incidence rate from 2004 to 2008, particularly in Hong Kong, Finland, the UK, Australia, the Netherlands, New Zealand, and Norway. Denmark was the only country with a significant increase in incidence, which was found to be higher in females.[48]

There is no known association of sinonasal cancer with any certain race or geographic region. Regarding etiology, unlike most other cancers of the head and neck, there has only been mild associations between tobacco and sinonasal tumors.[48] The main factor noted to be associated with sinonasal tumors is occupational exposure to wood dust from jobs in the wood-related industry, as well as other dusts in the leather/textiles industries.[51,52] Additionally, industrial exposure to certain minerals and chemicals (ie, nickel, chromium, cadmium, radium-226, radium-228, and formaldehyde) has been associated with sinonasal tumors.[48] HPV has also been implicated as being associated, given an HPV prevalence of 27% of patients with sinonasal tumors in a meta-analysis, but no causation has been proven.[53] Interestingly, there has been a decreasing trend in the occupational exposure of wood dust in most countries after wood dust was confirmed as a human carcinogen, possibly playing a role in the generalized decrease in sinonasal cancer incidence.[48]

In summary, the incidence and global burden of sinonasal cancers has fortunately been down trending in almost all studied countries, with the exception of Denmark. Emphasis should continue to be placed on tobacco cessation counseling as well as appropriate protection from occupational wood dust exposure (and other mineral/chemical exposures) to continue the trend of decreasing the global burden of sinonasal cancers.

DISCLOSURE

The authors have nothing to disclose.

REFERENCES

1. Jemal A, Bray F, Center MM, et al. Global cancer statistics. CA Cancer J Clin 2011;61(2):69–90.
2. Fidler MM, Bray F, Soerjomataram I. The global cancer burden and human development: a review. Scand J Public Health 2018;46(1):27–36.
3. Fidler MM, Soerjomataram I, Bray F. A global view on cancer incidence and national levels of the human development index. Int J Cancer 2016;139(11): 2436–46.
4. Ferlay J, Soerjomataram I, Dikshit R, et al. Cancer incidence and mortality worldwide: sources, methods and major patterns in GLOBOCAN 2012. Int J Cancer 2015;136(5):E359–86.
5. Du M, Nair R, Jamieson L, et al. Incidence trends of lip, oral cavity, and pharyngeal cancers: global burden of disease 1990-2017. J Dent Res 2019; 99(2):143–51.

6. Bray F, Ferlay J, Soerjomataram I, et al. Global cancer statistics 2018: GLOBOCAN estimates of incidence and mortality worldwide for 36 cancers in 185 countries. CA Cancer J Clin 2018;68(6): 394–424.

7. Chaturvedi AK, Anderson WF, Lortet-Tieulent J, et al. Worldwide trends in incidence rates for oral cavity and oropharyngeal cancers. J Clin Oncol 2013; 31(36):4550–9.

8. Franceschi S, Bidoli E, Herrero R, et al. Comparison of cancers of the oral cavity and pharynx worldwide: etiological clues. Oral Oncol 2000;36(1): 106–15.

9. Li YC, Ann-Joy Cheng, Li-Yu Lee, et al. Multifaceted mechanisms of areca nuts in oral carcinogenesis: the molecular pathology from precancerous condition to malignant transformation. J Cancer 2019; 10(17):4054–62.

10. Perry BJ, Zammit AP, Lewandowski AW. Sites of origin of oral cavity cancer in nonsmokers vs smokers: possible evidence of dental trauma carcinogenesis and its importance compared with human papillomavirus. JAMA Otolaryngol Head Neck Surg 2015;141(1):5–11.

11. Ram H, Sarkar J, Kumar H, et al. Oral cancer: risk factors and molecular pathogenesis. J Maxillofac Oral Surg 2011;10(2):132–7.

12. McCoy GD. A biochemical approach to the etiology of alcohol related cancers of the head and neck. Laryngoscope 1978;88(1 Pt 2 Suppl 8):59–62.

13. Blank M, Deshpande L, Balster RL. Availability and characteristics of betel products in the U.S. J Psychoactive Drugs 2008;40(3):309–13.

14. Lu CT, Yen YY, Ho CS, et al. A case-control study of oral cancer in Changhua County, Taiwan. J Oral Pathol Med 1996;25(5):245–8.

15. Gupta N, Gupta R, Acharya AK, et al. Changing trends in oral cancer - a global scenario. Nepal J Epidemiol 2016;6(4):613–9.

16. Johnson NW, Amarasinghe HK. Epidemiology and aetiology of head and neck cancers. In: Bernier J, editor. Head and neck cancer: multimodality management. 2nd edition. Springer: Springer; 2011. p. 1–57.

17. GLOBOCAN 2012: Estimated Cancer Incidence, Mortality and Prevalence Worldwide in 2012. [cited 2016 July 16].

18. Warnakulasuriya S. Global epidemiology of oral and oropharyngeal cancer. Oral Oncol 2009;45(4–5): 309–16.

19. Devins KM, Tetzlaff MT, Baloch Z, et al. The evolving landscape of HPV-related neoplasia in the head and neck. Hum Pathol 2019;94:29–39.

20. Andersen AS, Koldjaer Sølling AS, Ovesen T, et al. The interplay between HPV and host immunity in head and neck squamous cell carcinoma. Int J Cancer 2014;134(12):2755–63.

21. Bruni L, Diaz M, Castellsagué X, et al. Cervical human papillomavirus prevalence in 5 continents: meta-analysis of 1 million women with normal cytological findings. J Infect Dis 2010;202(12):1789–99.

22. Serrano B, Brotons M, Bosch FX, et al. Epidemiology and burden of HPV-related disease. Best Pract Res Clin Obstet Gynaecol 2018;47:14–26.

23. Sandulache VC, Wilde DC, Sturgis EM, et al. A Hidden Epidemic of "Intermediate Risk" Oropharynx Cancer. Laryngoscope Investig Otolaryngol 2019;4(6):617–23.

24. Garnaes E, Kiss K, Andersen L, et al. A high and increasing HPV prevalence in tonsillar cancers in Eastern Denmark, 2000-2010: the largest registry-based study to date. Int J Cancer 2015;136(9): 2196–203.

25. Garnaes E, Kiss K, Andersenet L, et al. Increasing incidence of base of tongue cancers from 2000 to 2010 due to HPV: the largest demographic study of 210 Danish patients. Br J Cancer 2015;113(1): 131–4.

26. Hwang TZ, Hsiao JR, Tsai CR, et al. Incidence trends of human papillomavirus-related head and neck cancer in Taiwan, 1995-2009. Int J Cancer 2015;137(2):395–408.

27. Shin A, Jung YS, Jung KW, et al. Trends of human papillomavirus-related head and neck cancers in Korea: national cancer registry data. Laryngoscope 2013;123(11):E30–7.

28. Brotherton JML, Bloem PN. Population-based HPV vaccination programmes are safe and effective: 2017 update and the impetus for achieving better global coverage. Best Pract Res Clin Obstet Gynaecol 2018;47:42–58.

29. Dilley S, Miller KM, Huh WK. Human papillomavirus vaccination: ongoing challenges and future directions. Gynecol Oncol 2020;156(2):498–502.

30. Lehtinen M, Paavonen J, Wheeler CM, et al. Overall efficacy of HPV-16/18 AS04-adjuvanted vaccine against grade 3 or greater cervical intraepithelial neoplasia: 4-year end-of-study analysis of the randomised, double-blind PATRICIA trial. Lancet Oncol 2012;13(1):89–99.

31. Kjaer SK, Sigurdsson K, Iversen OE, et al. A pooled analysis of continued prophylactic efficacy of quadrivalent human papillomavirus (Types 6/11/16/18) vaccine against high-grade cervical and external genital lesions. Cancer Prev Res (Phila) 2009; 2(10):868–78.

32. Cocchio S, Baldovin T, Bertoncello C, et al. Decline in hospitalization for genital warts in the Veneto region after an HPV vaccination program: an observational study. BMC Infect Dis 2017;17(1):249.

33. Guerra FM, Rosella LC, Dunn S, et al. Early impact of Ontario's human papillomavirus (HPV) vaccination program on anogenital warts (AGWs): A population-based assessment. Vaccine 2016; 34(39):4678–83.

34. Bollerup S, Baldur-Felskov B, Blomberg M, et al. Significant Reduction in the Incidence of Genital Warts in Young Men 5 Years into the Danish Human Papillomavirus Vaccination Program for Girls and Women. Sex Transm Dis 2016;43(4):238–42.

35. Lurie S, Mizrachi Y, Chodick G, et al. Impact of quadrivalent human papillomavirus vaccine on genital warts in an opportunistic vaccination structure. Gynecol Oncol 2017;146(2):299–304.

36. Chaturvedi AK, D'Souza G, Gillison ML, et al. Burden of HPV-positive oropharynx cancers among ever and never smokers in the U.S. population. Oral Oncol 2016;60:61–7.

37. Li K, Lin GZ, Shen JC, et al. Time trends of nasopharyngeal carcinoma in urban Guangzhou over a 12-year period (2000-2011): declines in both incidence and mortality. Asian Pac J Cancer Prev 2014;15(22): 9899–903.

38. Young LS, Dawson CW. Epstein-Barr virus and nasopharyngeal carcinoma. Chin J Cancer 2014;33(12): 581–90.

39. Bei JX, Li Y, Jia WH, et al. A genome-wide association study of nasopharyngeal carcinoma identifies three new susceptibility loci. Nat Genet 2010;42(7): 599–603.

40. Argirion I, Zarins KR, Ruterbusch JJ, et al. Increasing incidence of Epstein-Barr virus-related nasopharyngeal carcinoma in the United States. Cancer 2020;126(1):121–30.

41. Zhang B, Li MM, Chen WH, et al. Association of chemoradiotherapy regimens and survival among patients with nasopharyngeal carcinoma: a systematic review and meta-analysis. JAMA Netw Open 2019;2(10):e1913619.

42. Petersen JF, Timmermans AJ, van Dijk BAC, et al. Trends in treatment, incidence and survival of hypopharynx cancer: a 20-year population-based study in the Netherlands. Eur Arch Otorhinolaryngol 2018;275(1):181–9.

43. Bradley PJ, Eckel HE. Epidemiology of Hypopharyngeal cancer. Adv Otorhinolaryngol. Basel, Karger 2019;83:1–14.

44. Hochfelder CG, McGinn AP, Mehta V, et al. Treatment sequence and survival in locoregionally advanced hypopharyngeal cancer: a surveillance, epidemiology, and end results-based study. Laryngoscope 2019. [Epub ahead of print].

45. Zuniga SA, Lango MN. Effect of rural and urban geography on larynx cancer incidence and survival. Laryngoscope 2018;128(8):1874–80.

46. Iocca O, Farcomeni A, Di Rocco A, et al. Locally advanced squamous cell carcinoma of the head and neck: a systematic review and Bayesian network meta-analysis of the currently available treatment options. Oral Oncol 2018;80:40–51.

47. Cramer JD, Burtness B, Ferris RL. Immunotherapy for head and neck cancer: recent advances and future directions. Oral Oncol 2019;99:104460.

48. Youlden DR, Cramb SM, Peters S, et al. International comparisons of the incidence and mortality of sinonasal cancer. Cancer Epidemiol 2013;37(6):770–9.

49. Turner JH, Reh DD. Incidence and survival in patients with sinonasal cancer: a historical analysis of population-based data. Head Neck 2012;34(6): 877–85.

50. Dutta R, Dubal PM, Svider PF, et al. Sinonasal malignancies: a population-based analysis of site-specific incidence and survival. Laryngoscope 2015; 125(11):2491–7.

51. Gordon I, Boffetta P, Demers PA. A case study comparing a meta-analysis and a pooled analysis of studies of sinonasal cancer among wood workers. Epidemiology 1998;9(5):518–24.

52. WHO. Wood Dust. IARC Monogr Eval Carcinog Risks Hum 1995;(62):35–7.

53. Syrjanen K, Syrjanen S. Detection of human papillomavirus in sinonasal carcinoma: systematic review and meta-analysis. Hum Pathol 2013;44(6):983–91.

View from the Other Side: A Perspective on Oral and Maxillofacial Surgery in a Developing Nation - Bangladesh

Motiur Rahman Molla, BDS, PhD, FCPS, Dip – OMS, FICS, FICD[a],
Hussein K. Haji, BSc Pharm, RPh, DDS[b], Nafisa Marium Molla, BDS, DDS[c],*

KEYWORDS

- Dentistry • Oral surgery • Oral and maxillofacial surgery • Developing countries • Southeast Asia
- Bangladesh • India • Pakistan

KEY POINTS

- Substances shown to be potentially carcinogenic such as paan and betel nut are widely used in developing countries in Southeast Asia.
- Oral and maxillofacial surgeons in Southeast Asia often utilize diagnostic modalities including biopsy, histopathologic examination, computed tomography scanning, and magnetic resonance imaging.
- Oral and maxillofacial surgeons in the region routinely engage in head and neck oncological surgical cases, temporomandibular joint reconstructive procedures, and maxillofacial reconstructive surgeries.
- Foreign assistance allows maxillofacial surgeons in developing nations to advance their surgical skills and continue to provide optimal patient care.

INTRODUCTION

The evolution of oral and maxillofacial surgery in developing countries within Southeast Asia, such as Bangladesh, India, Pakistan, and Nepal, has been a multifaceted and challenging journey but has been productive and truly promising.

Initially, the field of maxillofacial surgery focused primarily on extraction of third molars and other simple surgical procedures but has steadily developed into an expansive practice involving a variety of surgical practices, including head and neck cancer, facial bone fractures, jaw cysts and tumors, oncological surgery with flap procedures and comprehensive reconstructions, dental implants, orthognathic surgery, full mouth rehabilitation, and others. At this point in time, with the use of paan, betel nut, betel quid, smokeless tobacco, and other potentially carcinogenic substances becoming more widespread and mainstream, cases involving advanced head and neck cancer are becoming a primary focus of oral and maxillofacial surgeons within these developing countries. Although the surgeries are advanced and comprehensive in nature and the community of surgeons has developed and expanded their repertoire of abilities and skills, assistance from the global community of oral and maxillofacial surgeons is welcomed and highly

[a] Department of Oral and Maxillofacial Surgery, Anwer Khan Modern Medical College and Hospital, Road-08, House-17, Dhanmondi, Dhaka 1207, Bangladesh; [b] 8 Minorca Place, Toronto, Ontario M3A 2Z6, Canada; [c] 1236, 125 Omni Drive, Toronto, Ontario M1P 5A9, Canada
* Corresponding author.
E-mail address: moti.molla@gmail.com

Oral Maxillofacial Surg Clin N Am 32 (2020) 377–388
https://doi.org/10.1016/j.coms.2020.04.008

appreciated. Current challenges faced by lower-middle–income countries, such as Bangladesh, India, Nepal, Pakistan, and others, include lack of awareness and late presentation in combination with inadequate access to surgical care, human resources, infrastructure, and equipment, with a growing need for sustainable initiatives in collaboration with the global community of oral and maxillofacial surgeons.

DEMOGRAPHICS

For the current 2020 fiscal year, according to the World Bank data, a gross national income per capita of $1025 or less in 2018 indicates low income, whereas that of $1026 to $3995 indicates lower-middle income. Countries with lower-middle–income economies include Bangladesh, India, Pakistan, Bhutan, and others.[1]

Bangladesh, India, and Nepal are similar in terms of demographics. In Bangladesh, the population growth rate was 1.1% in 2018, Nepal was 1.7%, and India 1.0%.[2] The birth rate in Bangladesh was 19 births per 1000 people in 2017, with a life expectancy of 72 years in 2017.[3,4]

The infant mortality rate in Bangladesh was 32.4 per 1000 live births in 2017.[5] In addition, the gross domestic product per capita in Bangladesh was recorded as $1203.20 in 2018.[6]

According to the World Bank, among South Asian countries, Bangladesh ranks second to last in terms of doctor-patient ratio, 0.5 per 1000 (2018), in comparison to India (0.8 in 2017), Pakistan (1.0 in 2015), Nepal (0.7 in 2017), and Sri Lanka (1.0 in 2017).[7]

SANITATION AND BASIC ORAL HYGIENE

Developing countries within Southeast Asia continue to have significant issues with sanitation, hygiene, pollution, and quality-of-life standards. These issues have resulted in tremendous health care challenges, including the widespread occurrence of diseases, both communicable and non-communicable. Worldwide health care organizations have studied and produced reports on the current sanitation and hygiene practices within these developing countries.

UNICEF has reported that although a developing country, such as Bangladesh, has made remarkable progress with respect to sanitation standards, there still is a considerable amount of improvement that must be made. The organization notes that "the knowledge of key hygiene messages is high in Bangladesh, but the practice of effective handwashing, the most effective hygiene behavior, is low."[8] The presence of sanitation is lacking most significantly among the poorest and most impoverished populations in Bangladesh.

Similarly, in India, sanitation, potable water, and hygiene practices are significantly lacking. UNICEF estimates that, to date, only a quarter of India's population has access to potable drinking water on premises. Moreover, more than 50% of the population defecates in the open and does not have access to proper hygiene facilities. This, in combination with widespread pollution and poor sanitation practices, has led to a high prevalence and occurrence of diseases, such as diarrhea, cholera, typhoid, respiratory infections, and skin and eye infections in India.

With respect to oral hygiene practices in developing Southeast Asian countries, common practices have included brushing with digits covered with charcoal or snuff or, alternatively, brushing with bare miswak sticks. This has transitioned slowly into the use of conventional toothbrushes and toothpaste, as awareness around oral hygiene and oral health continues to increase.

NUTRITIONAL DEFICIENCIES

The burden of nutritional deficiencies in Southeast Asia is considerable, especially among the female and pediatric populations. The World Health Organization estimates that underdeveloped countries in Southeast Asia account for more than 70% of malnourished children globally.[9] Among the different vitamin and mineral deficiencies prevalent in the region, iron deficiency and vitamin A deficiency are among those most commonly found.[9] It has been estimated that a significant proportion of school-aged children in Bangladesh possess deficiencies of vitamin A, zinc, vitamin D, and iron.[10] The regional practice of overboiling vegetables and food products before consumption, followed by discarding vitamin-rich and mineral-rich broth, also has been thought to be a contributing factor to nutritional deficiencies.

ANTIBIOTIC RESISTANCE

Antibiotic resistance is highly prevalent in developing countries in Southeast Asia. Resistance rates vary significantly, but all are cause of concern and alarm. A recent study focusing on antibiotic resistance in India revealed a concerning level of resistance to different pathogenic microbial organisms. For example, the study found more than 70% of *Klebsiella pneumoniae* bacteria and *Escherichia coli* bacteria, as well as almost half of *Pseudomonas aeruginosa* bacteria, displayed resistance to fluoroquinolone and third-generation cephalosporin antibiotics.[11] Similarly, a systematic review from 2019 focusing on antibiotic resistance in Bangladesh found that most pathogens displayed high levels of antibiotic resistance, and common first-line antimicrobial therapies generally were ineffective under most circumstances.[12] It has been hypothesized that the high levels of antimicrobial resistance most likely are due to the overuse and misuse of antimicrobial therapies, especially because they commonly are prescribed for simple therapies, such as dental prophylaxis and simple extractions.

THE PREVALENCE OF CANCER IN SOUTHEAST ASIA

In general, cancer is a common disease in different parts of Southeast Asia, including in India, Bangladesh, Pakistan, and Nepal; 86% of all oral cancer cases are reported to originate within India.[13] Breast cancer and cervical cancer are prevalent types of cancer found among Indian patients. In Bangladesh, oropharyngeal cancer and lung cancer have been found the most prevalent types of cancer afflicting Bangladeshi men, whereas cervical, uterine, and breast cancers are the most prevalent types of cancer affecting women in Bangladesh.[14]

With respect to head and neck cancer statistics, it has been reported that 30% of all malignancies in Southeast Asia are those of the head and neck region, whereas in Bangladesh it is reported to be 20%. In stark contrast to these statistics, the United Kingdom and the United States report that head and neck cancer cases comprise 2% to 7% of all oncological cases.[15]

In contrast to the distribution of common types of cancer in developing countries in Southeast Asia, developed countries, such as the United States, display higher prevalence rates of female breast and prostate cancers.[16] It is highly likely that the difference in regional cancer type distributions is due to the disparity in the prevalence of different risk factors for cancer occurrence, for example, the prevalence of use of different carcinogenic substances, such as tobacco, paan, betel nut, and quid.

THE WIDESPREAD USE OF CARCINOGENIC SUBSTANCES IN SOUTHEAST ASIA

A significant concern in India, Bangladesh, and other developing countries in Southeast Asia is the widespread and growing use of paan, betel nut, betel quid, and smokeless tobacco, substances that have been shown to possess potentially carcinogenic effects (**Fig. 1**). The use of these substances is prevalent in these countries,

and they typically are associated with cultural norms and standard household practices. One particular common regional practice employed by individuals and associated with high rates of leukoplakia and oral submucous fibrosis is parking snuff tobacco in the buccal mucosal area.

Although these potentially carcinogenic substances are well integrated into Southeast Asian culture, consumers and the average population largely are unaware of the carcinogenic and damaging effects that these substances can have on health and wellbeing. Consequently, patients typically present to general dentists and oral surgeons for general examinations or with minor concerns, only to learn that they possess pathologies, such as leukoplakia, oral submucous fibrosis, squamous cell carcinoma, and, in most cases, the most advanced forms of these pathologies. These patients often require surgical interventions and major reconstructive surgeries for stages 3 and 4 carcinomas with lymph node involvement.

Often, however, before presenting to hospitals and medical clinics, patients, especially those in rural areas, first receive homeopathic therapy in combination with vitamins, antibiotics, and other ineffective forms of therapy. The patients, after experiencing therapeutic failures, then are referred to general dental practitioners and dental specialists who then are able to guide patients toward more appropriate care. By the time patients present to an oral and maxillofacial surgeon, even with comprehensive surgical and multimodality treatment, they possess a poor prognosis and experience high recurrence rates. On average, in Bangladesh, oral and maxillofacial surgeons diagnosing and treating oropharyngeal squamous cell carcinoma have estimated prevalence rates of 20% to 30% for stages 1 and 2 carcinoma and 60% to 70% prevalence rates for stages 3 and 4 carcinoma.[17–19]

A HISTORY OF ORAL AND MAXILLOFACIAL SURGERY IN BANGLADESH

The field of oral and maxillofacial surgery was introduced formally in Bangladesh by Dr Motiur Rahman Molla in late 1980s, upon returning from his oral and maxillofacial surgery residency program and receiving his PhD in Japan (**Fig. 2**). The practice of surgery began at Dhaka Dental College and Hospital (DDC) with impacted third molar surgical extractions, enucleations, neoplastic surgeries, maxillofacial fracture management, and others. At the time, Dr. Rafique Ahmed Bhuiyan, Dr. S. M. Iqbal Shaheed, and Dr. Kh. Altaf Hossain,

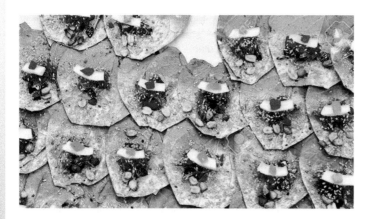

Fig. 1. Paan, a commonly consumed and potentially carcinogenic substance in Southeast Asia.

all internationally trained surgeons, were working with Dr. Molla. After a few years, Dr. Mohiuddin Ahmed, also an internationally trained surgeon educated in Japan, also joined the institution. At that time, extraction as a mode of therapy for decayed and unrestorable teeth was the treatment of choice, because endodontic therapy was not widely practiced or accepted. The use of the knowledge, skills, and experience gained from abroad contributed to not only patient care but also patient education. Endodontic therapy was introduced and promoted alongside surgical therapy, and patients were educated as to the value of oral hygiene and the maintenance of the dentition through endodontic therapy and comprehensive restorative work. In addition, experience from abroad encouraged the promotion and development of the other dental specialties, including periodontics, prosthodontics, anesthesia, orthodontics, and dental public health. Perhaps most significantly, oral surgeons and general dentists became more aware of the significant sanitation and oral hygiene–related issues in Bangladesh, and they began to counsel their patients more frequently on the value of exceptional oral hygiene, maintaining proper sanitation standards, and maintaining a healthy dentition and periodontium.

In 1994, in partnership with foreign maxillofacial surgeons from Australia and Japan, the University of Dhaka introduced the first master's degree program in oral and maxillofacial surgery in Bangladesh (**Fig. 3**). Dr. Rezaul Haq also joined the institution. The program's aim was to train and produce competent and exceptional native surgeons, with a comprehensive aptitude for oral and maxillofacial surgical procedures. The goal was to encourage Bangladeshi candidates to train in the specialty within Dhaka and serve the needs of the general population. In order to comprehensively prepare candidates, the residency in oral and maxillofacial surgery was assigned a length of 4 years, during which candidates underwent 6 months of training in general surgery; 3 months of ear, nose, and throat surgical training; 3 months of training in plastic and reconstructive surgery; 3 months of trauma surgery; 3 months in general medicine; and the remainder of the program training in oral and maxillofacial surgery. The program also requires candidates to complete a dissertation in order to achieve a fellowship or master of science degree in oral and maxillofacial surgery. To achieve licensure, candidates must pass oral examinations conducted by 4 qualified examiners, a panel usually consisting of 2 oral and maxillofacial surgeons, 1 general surgeon, and 1 foreign examiner.

Moreover, the master of science degree program received considerable assistance from Australian and Japanese oral and maxillofacial surgeons through educational partnerships with institutions from the 1990s to early 2000s (**Figs. 4 and 5**). During this time, Australian maxillofacial surgeons provided local surgeons with training on temporomandibular joint (TMJ) ankylosis surgery, treatment of facial bone fractures, simple autogenous bone reconstruction procedures, and management of jaw tumors, cysts, and other pathologies. Similarly, oral and maxillofacial surgeons from the Japanese Cleft Palate Foundation routinely visited Dhaka and other parts of Bangladesh primarily to lend their skills and talents to the treatment of both adult and pediatric patients suffering from cleft lip and palate congenital conditions. During that period of time, Bangladesh possessed a large number of patients with untreated cleft lip and palate.

From the aforementioned international educational collaborations, oral and maxillofacial surgeons in Bangladesh were able to utilize more

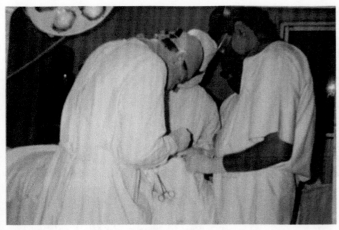
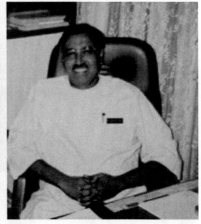

Fig. 2. Dr. Motiur Rahman Molla, pictured at the early stages of oral and maxillofacial surgery in Bangladesh, in both panels.

effectively the 20-bed maxillofacial surgical inpatient service department at DDC. In addition to cleft lip and palate patients, this inpatient service routinely treated patients suffering from TMJ ankylosis, maxillary and mandibular bony cysts and tumors, and a plethora of odontogenic and maxillofacial infections, including several cases of Ludwig angina. At that time, due to newly developing surgical sanitation principles and guidelines, as well as due to a lack of resources, many patients succumbed to their conditions, adding to a mortality rate that has been reduced considerably in modern times.

To further enhance the education of residents in the oral and maxillofacial surgery master's program, the governing professors and leadership at Dhaka Medical College and Hospital elected for the students to complete rotations in the ear, nose and throat; plastic surgery; casualty; emergency; and general surgery departments. By doing

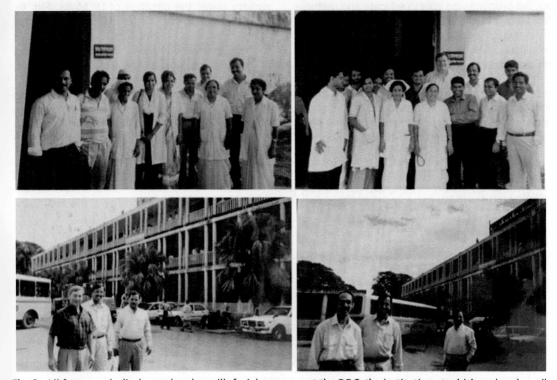

Fig. 3. All four panels display oral and maxillofacial surgeons at the DDC, the institution at which oral and maxillofacial surgery was introduced to the country.

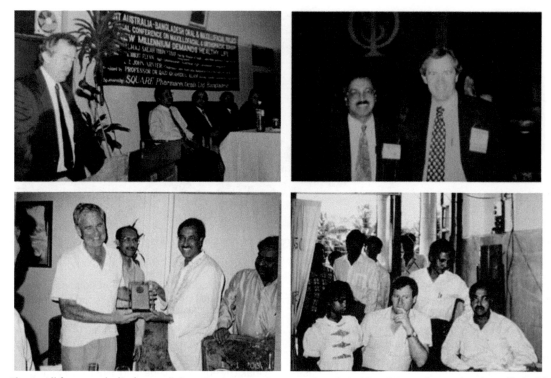

Fig. 4. All four panels display a collaborative initiative between Bangladeshi and Australian oral and maxillofacial surgeons.

so, the program was able to educate and matriculate surgeons with holistic and comprehensive surgical skills, prepared with the knowledge and experience needed to treat the diverse Bangladeshi population.

At Shaheed Suhrawardy Hospital, there initially was no in-patient service for oral surgery except for basic dentoalveolar procedures. In 2000, however, a new 18-bed in patient facility and an operating room was created for oral and maxillofacial surgery under the direction of Dr Molla (**Fig. 6**). Thus, the facility was better able to render a full range of oral and maxillofacial surgical services to the general populace. Between 2002 and 2003, DDC created a new campus in Mirpur, Bangladesh facilitating the beginning of a revolutionary 200-bed in-patient hospital (**Fig. 7**). The hospital divided the in-patient beds between an oral and maxillofacial surgical service (100 beds), general surgical service (50 beds), and the

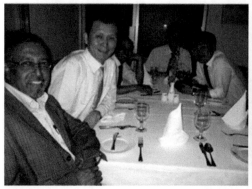

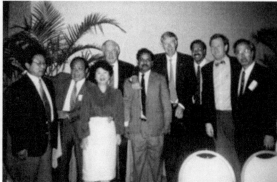

Fig. 5. Both panels display Collaborative initiatives between Bangladeshi, Japanese, and South Korean oral and maxillofacial surgeons.

Fig. 6. Shaheed Suhrawardy Hospital.

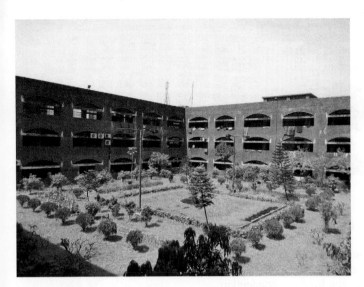

medicine service (50 beds). This new institution allowed for and promoted a further awareness of maxillofacial surgery in Bangladesh, and it serviced facilitating the care of patients suffering from head and neck diseases, such as head and neck pathology, intraoral cancers, and maxillofacial infections.

Until 2003, Dr. Al Mamoon Ferdousi, a foreign trained surgeon, coordinated the oral and maxillofacial surgical residency training program at Bangabandhu Sheikh Mujib Medical University (BSMMU). In 2004, Dr. Motiur Molla coordinated the opening of a 20-bed in-patient facility for oral surgery and an operating room for oral surgical procedures at BSMMU (**Fig. 8**). At this time, the oral and maxillofacial surgical residency training

program was revised in order to enhance the standards and requirements of the program.

As time progressed, there was a strong shift in the diversity of cases commonly seen by maxillofacial surgeons in Bangladesh. Initially, during the 1990s and early 2000s, surgeons commonly encountered cases involving head and neck infections, cellulitis, Ludwig angina, TMJ ankylosis, and cleft lip and palate. During the later 2000s, there was a shift toward a larger focus on head and neck cancer patients, patients with advanced jaw tumors, and those suffering from severe malocclusions requiring orthognathic surgery. It has been postulated that this shift was due to increased awareness of oral hygiene and sanitation, increased availability and prevalence of

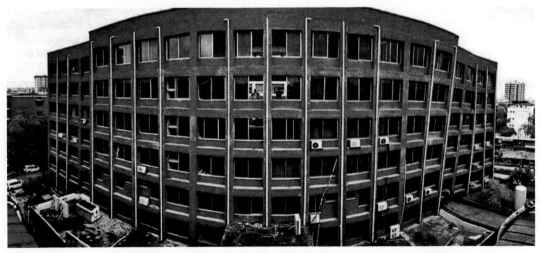

Fig. 7. DDC.

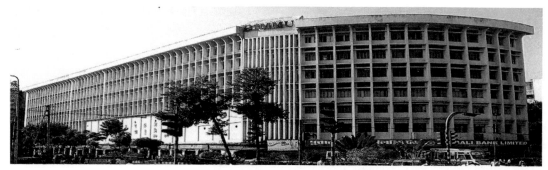

Fig. 8. BSMMU.

endodontics, and patients seeking care earlier and more expeditiously.

At the present time, the approximately 300 oral and maxillofacial surgeons who have matriculated from the master's and fellowship programs from both BSMMU and DDC focus on advanced head and neck surgical cancer cases, dental implant surgical procedures, orthognathic surgical cases, TMJ reconstructive procedures, and a continued practice mainly in reconstructive surgery with autogenous bone grafts, pedicle major flaps, and microvascular surgery. Bangladeshi trained oral and maxillofacial surgeons such as Dr. Ismat Ara Haider in collaboration with internationally trained surgeons such as Dr. Quazi Billur Rahman, a surgeon educated in the Soviet Union, continue to contribute significantly to the field of oral and maxillofacial surgery as it currently stands in Bangladesh.

Current Oral and Maxillofacial Surgical Practices in Southeast Asia

Head and neck cancer surgery and maxillofacial reconstruction

The prevalence of head and neck cancer, in particular squamous cell carcinoma, has increased since the advent of oral and maxillofacial surgery in Southeast Asia. This increase in prevalence most likely is due to an increased consumption and use of potentially carcinogenic substances, such as betel nut, betel quid, smokeless tobacco, and paan, as well as the high burden of human papillomavirus (HPV) in these developing countries. According to a 2009 survey by the World Health Organization, 23.5% of men and 25.2% of women over the age of 15 years in Bangladesh currently use or have used betel nut.[20] In India, the National Family Health Survey has estimated that 36.5% of men and 8.4% of women between the ages of 15 and 49 chew at least 1 type of tobacco.[21] Moreover, with respect to the burden of

HPV in Bangladesh, a recent research article by Shaikh and colleagues[22] found that 36% of oropharyngeal cancers, 31% of oral cancers, and 22% of laryngeal cancers were linked to HPV coinfection.

The increasing prevalence of head and neck cancer not only has had a negative impact on public health in these countries but also has had a significant macroeconomic impact. A 2015 study by Alkire and colleagues[23] has estimated that economic losses due to head and neck cancer in India, Pakistan, and Bangladesh in 2010 alone were approximately $16.9 billion, with Bangladesh experiencing the highest proportional losses.

With the rising burden of advanced head and neck cancers in developing Southeast Asian countries, in particular squamous cell carcinoma, oral and maxillofacial surgeons have refined and advanced their surgical treatment modalities and techniques. Modern surgical and diagnostic modalities are advanced and have high levels of accuracy and effectiveness. Oral and maxillofacial surgeons often utilize diagnostic modalities, including incisional and excisional biopsy, punch biopsy, fine-needle biopsy, microscopic histopathologic examination, computed tomography scan, magnetic resonance imaging, radionuclide scanning, and TNM staging systems.[24] The different therapeutic modalities used in the treatment of head and neck cancer patients also have advanced considerably since the introduction of maxillofacial surgery in Southeast Asia. Surgeons routinely perform resection procedures for head and neck tumors, accompanied by neck dissection procedures, and intraoperative frozen section biopsy, in order to confirm noncancerous margins.[24] Unlike in more developed countries, however, these resective procedures are followed by reconstruction, primarily using pedicle and regional flaps, including the temporalis flap, submental island flap, pectoralis major flap, and several others. This is an advancement over the historical use of stainless-steel plates with autogenous iliac bone graft for reconstruction surgery as well as the use of acrylic obturators primarily for maxillary postsurgical defects. Due to the current sheer volume of head and neck cancer cases, lengthy reconstructive procedures using microvascular grafts are less common, to date.

Dental implant surgery

Dental implant surgery was introduced to Bangladesh between 2003 and 2004 at BSMMU. During this time, a visiting oral and maxillofacial surgeon from South Korea presented on the topic of dental implants to the Bangladeshi oral and maxillofacial surgical community. In addition, implant companies and specialists from a variety of other countries, including the United States, Switzerland, India, and others, provided significant assistance in order to advance implant dentistry in Bangladesh. From that time onward, maxillofacial surgeons in Bangladesh have developed their implant surgical techniques in conjunction with the development and growth of dental implant companies in Bangladesh. Oral and maxillofacial surgeons and specialists in the field of dental implant surgery continue to provide training programs and lectures to encourage further involvement of the dental community in the provision of dental implants to patients as a mode of dental rehabilitation.

Temporomandibular joint surgery

At the onset of oral and maxillofacial surgery in Southeast Asia, surgeons noted the significant number of patients experiencing TMJ ankylosis. It was hypothesized at this time that the large number of cases was due to patients having experienced prior traumatic fractures, such as condylar fractures, and never seeking reparative treatment. Also, it was hypothesized further that the joint ankylosis may have been due to untreated middle ear infections, which had spread to the TMJs, resulting in subsequent ankylosis.

In 1996, Molla and Shrestha[25] published an analytical study focusing on TMJ ankylosis. At this time, oral and maxillofacial surgeons utilized condylectomy surgical procedures to treat ankylosis with temporalis muscle flaps or auricular cartilage to prevent reankylosis.[25] The study concluded that condylectomy with temporalis muscle flap was the best surgical therapy for TMJ ankylosis at the time.[25]

With respect to TMJ surgical reconstruction in Bangladesh, Dr. Quazi Billur Rahman, in cooperation with Dr. Molla and Dr. Mohammad Emranul Islam introduced and utilized the costochondral graft for reconstruction after bilateral condylectomy to release TMJ ankylosis in a pediatric patient.[26] This surgical procedure was met with success, and surgeons have continued to use this procedure for pediatric TMJ reconstructive procedures as well as the temporalis muscle flap for adult reconstructions.[25,26]

Bangladeshi oral and maxillofacial surgeons also have successfully utilized amniotic membrane in the surgical treatment and rehabilitation of TMJ ankylosis.[27] In a 2016 study conducted by Akhter and colleagues,[27] the researchers postulated that, based on the success of the amniotic membrane as an interpositional material, this would be a biocompatible and economical material that can utilized in surgical cases involving TMJ ankylosis.

Orthognathic surgery

To date, orthognathic surgery continues to have low acceptability and utilization in Southeast Asia. During the time when orthognathic surgery was introduced to these countries, oral and maxillofacial surgeons used fixation plates/wires constructed from stainless steel rather than titanium. The stainless-steel fixation plates were of poor quality and their use often was followed by infections and the need for subsequent removal within a few years. Slowly, as more surgeons practice orthognathic surgery in these countries, titanium plates and hardware are becoming more available for use, resulting in better treatment outcomes. Interdisciplinary care and treatment planning in conjunction with orthodontists for presurgical orthognathic evaluation and management continue, however, to be a challenge. In recent times, Bangladesh has an active collaboration with oral and maxillofacial surgeons in the United States in order to enhance the care of orthognathic patients (**Fig. 9**).

The Future of Oral and Maxillofacial Surgery in Southeast Asia

The field of oral and maxillofacial surgery has expanded rapidly and progressed in Southeast Asia since its introduction. Further progress and advancements are needed, however, in order to better enhance patient care, expand accessibility to care, and improve treatment outcomes (**Fig. 10**). For these goals to become a possibility, the oral and maxillofacial surgical community would benefit greatly from the voluntary involvement and intellectual contributions of oral and maxillofacial surgeons in developed countries, such as Canada, the United States, Australia, Japan, South Korea, and so forth. Foreign assistance, in any way possible, will allow maxillofacial surgeons in Southeast Asian developing countries, such as India, Bangladesh, Pakistan, and Nepal, to

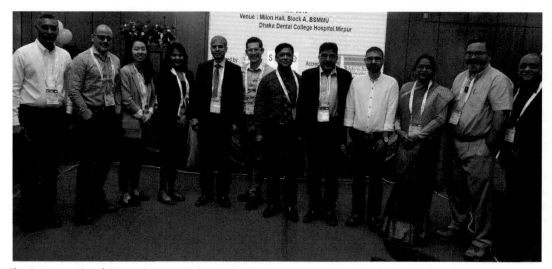

Fig. 9. International Symposium on Orthognathic Surgery.

enhance their surgical skills further and promote better patient care. The community welcomes all help, and any assistance always is appreciated.

Among various methods and strategies to enhance oral and maxillofacial surgery in developing Southeast Asian nations and to improve patient care and outcome, certain specific initiatives may prove the most productive and beneficial. In particular, rather than short local visits by foreign organizations and highly trained surgeons, longer periods of foreign didactic and clinical surgical training and research involvement for Southeast Asian surgical candidates may prove more beneficial in the long term. Moreover, additional collaborative efforts and educational connections between Southeast Asian and foreign training programs, such as those in Australia, Japan, and the United States, would prove effective. These educational collaborations would allow further enhancements and improvements to be made to local oral and maxillofacial surgical residency curricula and methods of standardized examination. Lastly, in addition to the remarkable value of educational enhancement, existing Southeast Asian oral and maxillofacial surgeons would highly benefit from improved access to modern surgical technologies and techniques, high-quality surgical materials such as titanium plates and screws for surgical procedures, and more stringent and regulated guidelines on infection control practices, and protocols, all of which may be facilitated by and supported by foreign institutions, surgeons, and organizations.

Supporting and enhancing the aforementioned objectives and goals is Smile Bangladesh, an American nonprofit medical organization committed to the treatment and support of both children and adults in Bangladesh living with orofacial cleft palate and facial cleft deformities. The organization, founded by Dr Shahid R. Aziz, provides complimentary care to these patients through the voluntary service of foreign surgeons, anesthesiologists, nurses, and other health care professionals (**Fig. 11**).[28]

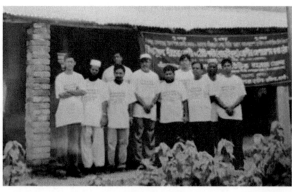
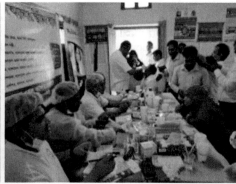

Fig. 10. Both panels display rural dental camps in Southeast Asia.

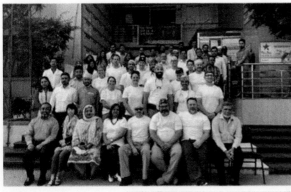
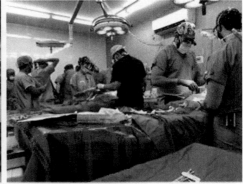
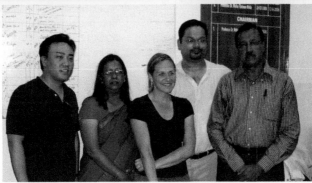

Fig. 11. All panels display Dr Shahid Aziz and the Smile Bangladesh initiative.

The future of oral and maxillofacial surgery in developing countries within Southeast Asia is promising and exciting. With technology, techniques, and education continually developing and expanding, the field of oral and maxillofacial surgery in Southeast Asia also can continue to develop and progress. This will, hopefully and overall, lead to enhanced patient care and better clinical patient outcomes.

DISCLOSURE

The authors have nothing to disclose.

REFERENCES

1. The World Bank Data. World Bank Country and Lending Groups. Available at: https://datahelpdesk.worldbank.org/knowledgebase/articles/906519-world-bank-country-and-lending-groups. Accessed October 10, 2019.
2. The World Bank Data. Population growth (annual %) – Bangladesh. Available at: https://data.worldbank.org/indicator/SP.POP.GROW?locations=BD. Accessed October 10, 2019.
3. The World Bank Data. Birth rate, crude (per 1,000 people) – Bangladesh. Available at: https://data.worldbank.org/indicator/SP.DYN.CBRT.IN?locations=BD. Accessed October 10, 2019.
4. The World Bank Data. Life expectancy at birth, total (years) – Bangladesh. Available at: https://data.worldbank.org/indicator/SP.DYN.LE00.IN?locations=BD. Accessed October 10, 2019.
5. Unicef Data. Key demographic indicators. Available at: https://data.unicef.org/country/bgd/. Accessed October 10, 2019.
6. The World Bank Data. GDP per capita (current US$)-Bangladesh. Available at: https://data.worldbank.org/indicator/NY.GDP.PCAP.CD?locations=BD. Accessed October 10, 2019.
7. The World Bank Data. Physicians (per 1,000 people). Available at: https://data.worldbank.org/indicator/sh.med.phys.zs. Accessed October 10, 2019.
8. Unicef Bangladesh. Safer sanitation and hygiene. Available at: https://www.unicef.org/bangladesh/en/better-access-safe-drinking-water/safer-sanitation-and-hygiene. Accessed October 12, 2019.
9. World Health Organization. Regional nutrition strategy: addressing malnutrition and micronutrient deficiencies (2011-2015). Available at: https://apps.who.int/iris/handle/10665/205804. Accessed October 12, 2019.
10. Ahmed F, Prendiville N, Narayan A. Micronutrient deficiencies among children and women in

Bangladesh: progress and challenges. J Nutr Sci 2016;5(46):1–12.

11. Taneja N, Sharma M. Antimicrobial resistance in the environment: The Indian scenario. Indian J Med Res 2019;149(2):119–28.

12. Ahmed I, Rabbi MB, Sultana S. Antibiotic resistance in Bangladesh: A systematic review. Int J Infect Dis 2019;80:54–61.

13. NICPR. These are the signs and symptoms of the most common types of cancer in India. Available at: http://cancerindia.org.in/signs-symptoms-common-types-cancer-india/. Accessed October 12, 2019.

14. Hussein SMA. Comprehensive update on cancer scenario of Bangladesh. South Asian J Cancer 2013;2(4):279–84.

15. Akhter M, Hossain S, Rahman QB, et al. A study on histological grading of oral squamous cell carcinoma and its co-relationship with regional metastasis. J Oral Maxillofac Pathol 2011;15(2):168–76.

16. U.S. Cancer Statistics Working Group. U.S. cancer statistics data visualizations tool, based on November 2018 submission data (1999-2016). U.S. Department of Health and Human Services, Centers for Disease Control and Prevention and National Cancer Institute; 2019. Available at: www.cdc.gov/cancer/dataviz. Accessed October 12, 2019.

17. Shaheed SMI, Molla MR. Oral cancer in Bangladesh: its etiology and histological grading. J Oral Health 1996;2:8–11.

18. Sadat SMS. Oral squamous cell carcinoma of Bangladeshi patients: a survival study. Int J Oral Maxillofac Surg 2013;42(10).

19. Uddin N, Iqbal M, Urmee FZ, et al. Factors influencing early recurrence of oral squamous cell

carcinoma – a study in a tertiary level hospital of Bangladesh. BJDRE 2018;8(1).

20. Fact Sheet Global Adult Tobacco Survey (GATS) Bangladesh. 2009. Available at: https://www.who.int/tobacco/surveillance/fact_sheet_of_gats_bangladesh_2009.pdf. Accessed October 11, 2019.

21. IARC Working Group on the Evaluation of Carcinogenic Risk to Humans. Personal Habits and Indoor Combustions. Lyon (FR): International Agency for Research on Cancer. 2012. Available at: https://www.ncbi.nlm.nih.gov/books/NBK304393. Accessed October 12, 2019.

22. Shaikh MH, Khan AI, Sadat A, et al. Prevalence and types of high-risk human papillomaviruses in head and neck cancers from Bangladesh. BMC Cancer 2017;17:792.

23. Alkire BC, Bergmark RW, Chambers K, et al. Head and neck cancer in South Asia: Macroeconomic consequences and the role of the head and neck surgeon. Head Neck 2016;38:1242–7. Wiley Periodicals, Inc.

24. Sultana J, Bashar A, Molla MR. New management strategies of oral tongue cancer in Bangladesh. J Maxillofac Oral Surg 2014;13(4):394–400.

25. Molla MR, Shrestha KR. An analytic study of surgical management of the temporomandibular joint ankylosis: an experience in Bangladesh. Bangladesh Med Res Counc Bull 1996;22(1):43–50.

26. Rahman QB, Molla MR, Islam ME. Temporomandibular joint reconstruction using costochondral graft. Mymensingh Med J 2007;16(2):225–9.

27. Akhter M, Ahmed N, Arefin MR, et al. Outcome of amniotic membrane as an interpositional arthroplasty of TMJ ankylosis. Oral Maxillofac Surg 2016;20(1):63–71.

28. Our Mission. Smile Bangladesh. Available at: http://www.smilebangladesh.org/our-mission.html. Accessed October 11, 2019.

Diversity and Cultural Competency in Oral and Maxillofacial Surgery

Jessica S. Lee, DDS, MD, MA[a], Shahid R. Aziz, DMD, MD, FRCS(Ed)[b,c,d,e],*

KEYWORDS

- Health disparity • Diversity • Race • Gender • Underrepresented minority • Cultural competency
- Humanitarian mission

KEY POINTS

- As the world becomes more diverse, it is imperative that the health care professional workforce is trained to care for the diversifying patient population.
- Improving the diversity within the health care professional workforce likely will aid in emphasizing the importance of cultural competency of health care professionals.
- Development of programs aimed at improving cultural competency of the health care professional workforce is necessary to meet the needs of a diverse patient population.

Health disparities in the United States have been well documented over the past several decades and continue to affect the American population today. The Centers for Disease Control and Prevention health disparities report in 2013 reported that non-Hispanic black adults in the Untied States are 50% more likely to die from heart disease or stroke prematurely (less than 75 years of age) than their non-Hispanic white counterparts.[1] The prevalence of diabetes also is higher among Hispanics, non-Hispanic blacks, and those of "other" or mixed races than that of Asians or non-Hispanic whites. Health disparities in the access of oral health care also exist within minorities groups, as reported in the first-ever Surgeon General report on oral health in America, published in 2000.[2] This report found that black patients were less likely to be diagnosed with localized oral or pharyngeal cancer than whites, stating that black patients were more likely to present to their dentist or physician with more advanced disease. More alarmingly, the report found that at every stage of diagnosis, the 5-year relative survival rates for blacks with oral and pharyngeal cancers were lower than that for whites.[2] Furthermore, the 5-year survival rates for blacks were found to be less than those of their white counterparts in almost all forms of cancer except gastric, brain, and pancreatic cancers and multiple myeloma. These statistics point to the health disparities that exist in the access to adequate and equal health care for minority groups within the United States.

These health disparities often are exacerbated by a lack of health care providers per person within minority communities compared with white communities, where safety net hospitals and clinics often form the bulk of providers. Furthermore, physicians who care for minority patients more often are overworked and underpaid compared with

a Pediatric Cleft and Craniofacial Surgery, Cleft and Craniofacial Surgery Center, Charleston Area Medical Center Women and Children's Hospital, 830 Pennsylvania Avenue, Suite 302, Charleston, WV 25302, USA; b Department of Oral and Maxillofacial Surgery, Rutgers School of Dental Medicine, Newark, NJ, USA; c Division of Plastic and Reconstructive Surgery, Department of Surgery, Rutgers – New Jersey Medical School, Newark, NJ, USA; d Update Dental College, Dhaka, Bangladesh; e Smile Bangladesh
* Corresponding author. Department of Oral and Maxillofacial Surgery, Rutgers School of Dental Medicine, 110 Bergen Street, Room B854, Newark, NJ 07103.
E-mail address: azizsr@sdm.rutgers.edu

Oral Maxillofacial Surg Clin N Am 32 (2020) 389–405
https://doi.org/10.1016/j.coms.2020.04.006
1042-3699/20/© 2020 Elsevier Inc. All rights reserved.

those who predominantly treat white patients.[3–5] These health disparities are exacerbated further by provision of low-quality care, with minorities lacking access to regular health care providers and often forced to resort to an emergency department, community health clinic, or hospital as their regular source of medical care.[6]

US POPULATION DEMOGRAPHICS

According to the US Census, in the year 2018, non-Hispanic whites comprised 60.4% of the 327,167,434 people in the US population.[7] Hispanics/Latinos represented 18.3% of the total US population, blacks 13.4%, Asians 5.9%, Native Americans/Alaska Natives 1.3%, and Native Hawaiians/Pacific Islanders 0.2% (**Fig. 1**).[7] As the world becomes more interconnected with the ease of travel, populations are becoming more diverse, composed of multiple races, ethnicities, cultures, and religions within a given geographic location. The United States is no exception: the US Census Bureau estimates that by the year 2044, more than half of all Americans are projected

to belong to a minority group (any group other than non-Hispanic white alone), and, by 2060, approximately 1 in 5 of the nation's total population is projected to be foreign born.[7]

US HEALTH CARE PROFESSIONAL RACIAL DEMOGRAPHICS
Racial Demographics in Medicine

The anticipated increase in diversity in the American population, however, does not correlate with the racial and ethnic demographics of health care professionals in training and the workforce. Racial demographics of US physicians in the workforce illustrate a disparity in which Hispanics and blacks are underrepresented. The Association of American Medical Colleges (AAMC) reported that of the total active US physicians in the year 2013, 48.9% were non-Hispanic white, 11.7% Asian, 4.4% Hispanic/Latino, 4.1% black/African American, and 0.4% American Indian/Alaska Native (**Fig. 2**).[8]

The lack of diversity in the US physician workforce likely is secondary to the lack of diversity

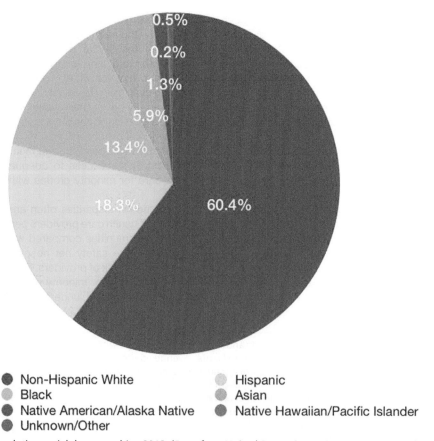

Fig. 1. US population racial demographics, 2018. (*Data from* United States Census Bureau. US census bureau quick facts: United States. 2018. Available at: https://www.census.gov/quickfacts/fact/table/US/PST045218.)

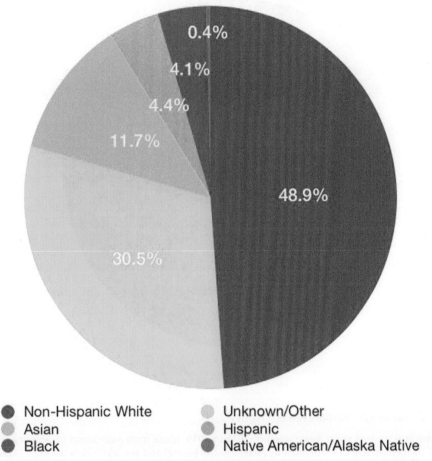

Non-Hispanic White   Unknown/Other
Asian   Hispanic
Black   Native American/Alaska Native

Fig. 2. US physician workforce racial demographics 2013. (*Data from* Association of American Medical Colleges. Diversity in the physician workforce: Facts & figures 2014. Available at: http://www.aamcdiversityfactsandfigures. org/section-ii-current-status-of-us-physician-workforce/index.html#fig1.)

found among students and residents in medical schools and in residency training programs. The AAMC reported that of the total 92,758 US medical students matriculated during the 2019 to 2020 academic year, 46,205 (49.8%) students were non-Hispanic white; 20,836 (22.5%) Asian; 6783 (7.3%) black; 6063 (6.5%) Hispanic/Latino; 199 (0.2%) Native American/Alaska Native; and 76 (0.1%) Native Hawaiian/Pacific Islander; and 12,596 (13.6%) identified as multiple/unknown ethnicity, non-US citizen/permanent resident, or other (**Fig. 3**).[9]

Representation of minority groups in leadership positions, namely medical school faculty, also paints a picture of underrepresentation. Of the total 175,889 full-time faculty during the 2018 to 2019 academic year, only 6331 (3.6%) were black/African American; 5691 (3.2%) Hispanic/Latino; 35,338 (19.5%) Asian; 276 (0.2%) Native American/Alaska Native; and 187 (0.1%) Native

Hawaiian/Pacific Islander; and 16,605 (9.4%) identified as other or multiple races, whereas the remaining 112,461 (64%) were non-Hispanic white (**Fig. 4**).[10] These statistics demonstrate that non-Hispanic whites and Asians are overrepresented in medicine, whereas blacks and Hispanics are underrepresented compared with the racial demographics of the US population.

Racial Demographics in Dentistry

Similar statistics of overrepresentation of non-Hispanic whites and Asians and underrepresentation of blacks and Hispanics also are demonstrated in dentistry, within dental schools, residency programs, and the workforce. The American Dental Association reported that of the 191,772 active US dentists in the workforce during the year 2016, 139,827 (73.6%) dentists were non-Hispanic white; 8182 (4.3%) black;

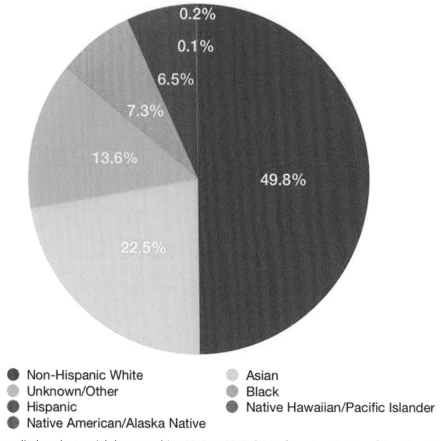

Fig. 3. US medical student racial demographics, 2018 to 2019. (*Data from* Association of American Medical Colleges. Total US medical school enrollment by race/ethnicity (alone) and sex, 2015-2016 through 2019-2020. Available at: https://www.aamc.org/system/files/2019-11/2019_FACTS_Table_B-3.pdf.)

10,040 (5.3%) Hispanic; and 30,089 (15.8%) Asian; and 1966 (1.0%) identified as other (**Fig. 5**).[11] The American Dental Association reported that of the 25,381 total US predoctoral dental students enrolled during the 2018 to 2019 academic year, there were 12,977 (51.1%) white students; 6099 (24%) Asian; 2293 (9.0%) Hispanic; 1338 (5.3%) black; 91 (0.4%) Native American/Alaska Native; and 54 (0.2%) Native Hawaiian/Pacific Islander students; and 2529 (10%) students who identified with 2 or more races or as nonresident aliens or were unknown (**Fig. 6**).[12] During the same academic year, there were a total of 7318 postgraduate US dental residents matriculated, of whom 3979 (54.4%) were white; 1687 (23.1%) were Asian; 628 (8.6%) were Hispanic; 315 (4.3%) were black; 21 (0.3%) were Native Hawaiian/Pacific Islander; and 13 (0.2%) were Native American/Alaska Native; and 675 (9.2%) identified with 2 or more races or a nonresident alien or were unknown (**Fig. 7**).[13]

Full-time US dental school faculty demonstrated a similar disparity in that among the 4867 full-time faculty in the 2016 to 2017 academic year; 2969 (61.0%) were white; 610 (12.5%) were Asian; 425 (8.7%) were Hispanic; 245 (5.0%) were black; 11 (0.2%) were Native American/Alaska Native; and 9 (0.2%) were Native Hawaiian/Pacific Islander; and 598 (12.3%) identified with 2 or more races or as nonresident alien or were unknown (**Fig. 8**).[14]

Racial Demographics in Oral and Maxillofacial Surgery

During the 2018 to 2019 academic year, there were a total of 1208 oral and maxillofacial surgery (OMS) residents enrolled, of whom 824 (68.2%) residents were white; 223 (18.5%) were Asian; 65 (5.4%) were Hispanic; 37 (3.1%) were black; 9 (0.7%) were Native Hawaiian/Pacific Islander; and 3 (0.2%) were Native American/Alaska Native; and 47 (3.9%) identified as 2 or more races or as nonresident alien, or unknown (**Fig. 9**).[15]

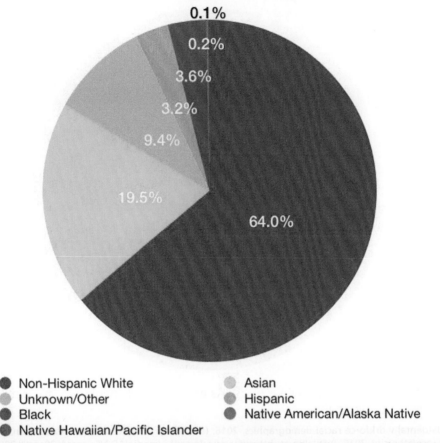

Fig. 4. US medical school full-time faculty racial demographics, 2018. (*Data from* Association of American Medical Colleges. US medical school faculty by sex and race/ethnicity, 2018. Available at: https://www.aamc.org/system/files/reports/1/18table8.pdf.)

During the 2019 to 2020 academic year, there were a total of 1118 OMS faculty affiliated with 101 accredited OMS programs in the United States and Puerto Rico, where 757 (67.7%) OMS faculty were white; 112 (10.0%) were Asian; 61 (5.5%) were Middle Eastern; 47 (4.2%) were black; 39 (3.5%) were Hispanic; 2 (0.2%) were Native American/Alaska Native; and 100 (8.9%) were other or unknown (American Association of Oral and Maxillofacial Surgery; 2019-2020 Faculty members summary report, Personal communication, 2019) (**Fig. 10**).

When analyzing the demographic makeup of those holding leadership positions in organized OMS, the disproportionate underrepresentation of minorities also is demonstrated. The American Association of Oral and Maxillofacial Surgeons (AAOMS) officers and trustees for 2019 to 2020 were composed of 12 (92.3%) white surgeons and 1 (7.7%) Hispanic surgeon.[16] The Board of Directors of the American Board of Oral and Maxillofacial Surgery (ABOMS) for 2019 to 2020 was composed of 6 (75%) white surgeons and 2 (25%) Asian surgeons.[17] The American College of Oral and Maxillofacial Surgeons (ACOMS) Board of Regents for 2019 to 2020 was composed of 7 (58.3%) white, 3 (25%) Hispanic, and 2 (16.7%) Asian surgeons.[18]

These statistics again demonstrate that non-Hispanic whites and Asians are overrepresented in dentistry and OMS, whereas blacks and Hispanics are underrepresented compared with the racial demographics of the total US population (**Fig. 11**).

US HEALTH CARE PROFESSIONAL GENDER DEMOGRAPHICS
Gender Demographics in Medicine

Representation of women has seen an appreciable progression in medicine. In 2017, there were approximately 800,300 physicians in the US workforce, where women constituted approximately one-third of physicians.[19] Of the 175,889

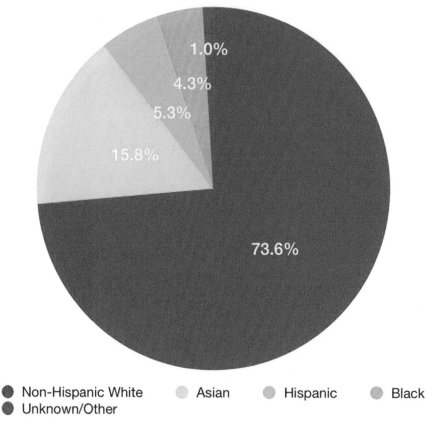

1.0%

4.3%

5.3%

15.8%

73.6%

● Non-Hispanic White   ● Asian   ● Hispanic   ● Black
● Unknown/Other

Fig. 5. US dental workforce racial demographics, 2016. (*Data* from American Dental Association. Dentist workforce by race/ethnicity, 2016. Available at: https://www.ada.org/~/media/ADA/Science%20and%20Research/HPI/Files/HPIData_Profile_2016.xlsx?la=en.)

US medical school faculty, 73,236 (41.7%) physicians were women.[10] During the 2017 to 2018 medical residency year, there were 58,965 (45.6%) women in training of the total 129,291 medical residents in the United States.[20] There were 46,878 women enrolled in medical school during the 2019 to 2020 academic year, constituting 50.5% of the 92,758 total US medical school enrollees, which has been on an upward trend over the past decade.[9] With this increase in representation of women in medical school and residency, more women are likely to enter the physician workforce, lending to an overall increase in representation of women in medicine.

Gender Demographics in Dentistry

In 2016, women represented less than one-third of the entire US dental workforce, making up 56,544 (29.5%) of the 135,228 total US dentists,[11] whereas 1890 (38.8%) of 4867 of full-time dental school faculty were women.[14] During the 2018 to 2019 academic year, 12,822 women were enrolled in dental school, constituting 50.5% of the 25,381

total US dental students (years 1 through 4), surpassing the proportion of men enrolled in dental school for the first time.[12]

Gender Demographics in Medical and Dental Postgraduate Training

As training advances within medical or dental residency and their subspecialties, representation of women begins to decrease, compared with that of medical or dental school. During the 2018 to 2019 academic year, for example, women represented 46.4% of the total US postgraduate dental residents (compared with women representing 50.5% of dental school students)[12,13] and 45.6% of the total US postgraduate medical residents during the 2017–2018 academic year (compared with women representing 49.5% of medical school students enrolled in 2019–2020).[9,20] Furthermore, a stark discrepancy of representation exists between men and women within specific medical and dental postgraduate subspecialties. In general, men tend to be overrepresented within the surgical subspecialties in medicine and dentistry,

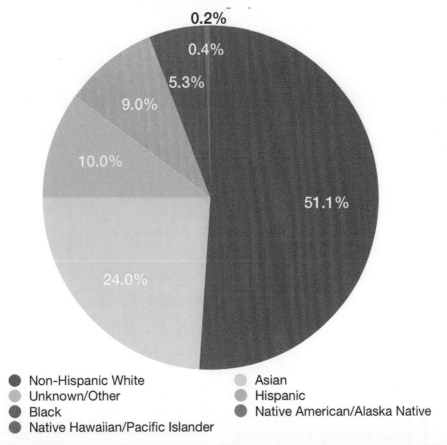

Fig. 6. Predoctoral dental student racial demographics, 2018 to 2019. (*Data from* American Dental Association. 2018-2019 Survey of dental education. Available at: https://www.ada.org/~/media/ADA/Science%20and%20Research/HPI/Files/SDE1_2018-19.xlsx?la=en.)

such as orthopedic surgery, neurosurgery, thoracic surgery, and OMS.[13,20] In contrast, women are overrepresented in the medical and dental subspecialties, such as obstetrics and gynecology, pediatrics, and pediatric dentistry (83.4%, 72.1%, and 67.1%, respectively).[20,21]

Gender Demographics in Oral and Maxillofacial Surgery

Women remain underrepresented in OMS and comprised only 16.2% of the OMS resident population in the United States during the 2019 to 2020 academic year.[13] Although this has been on an upward trend (15% women in 2014), representation of women in postgraduate dental training continues to be the lowest in the field of OMS, with the second lowest endodontics, which has more than double the percentage of women than that of OMS (16.2% vs 35.8%, respectively) (**Fig. 12**).[13,22] Furthermore, the increase in representation of female OMS residents over the years

has been outpaced by the increase in representation of female residents in similar surgical subspecialties, such as plastic and reconstructive surgery and otolaryngology (40.7% women and 35.6% women, respectively)[20,23] and ranks only second to orthopedic surgery (15.3%) in the least amount of female representation within a medical or dental surgical subspecialty (see **Fig. 12**; **Fig. 13**).

The representation of women in OMS postresidency is, staggeringly, even less than that of the representation of women within residency, with 565 (8%) of the 6700 registered AAOMS fellows in 2018 composed of women.[23] As expected, women also are underrepresented in organizational and academic OMS. Of the total 101 accredited OMS programs in the United States and Puerto Rico, a total of 20 women (19.8%) held a program director and/or chair position in the year 2019.[16] At the time of this publication, there was no woman serving as president in a major governing OMS organization, including AAOMS, ABOMS, and ACOMS.[16–18] Three (25%)

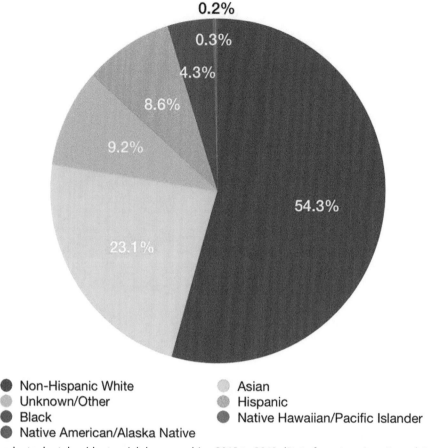

Fig. 7. Postgraduate dental resident racial demographics, 2018 to 2019. (*Data from* American Dental Association. 2018-2019 Survey of advanced dental education. Available at: https://www.ada.org/~/media/ADA/Science%20and%20Research/HPI/Files/SADV_2018-19.xlsx?la=en.)

of 12 surgeons serving on the 2019 to 2020 ACOMS Board of Regents were women and 1 (7.7%) of 13 surgeons serving on the 2019 to 2020 AAOMS Board of Trustees was a woman.[16,18] All 8 surgeons serving as 2018 to 2019 ABOMS Board of Directors were men.[17] At the time of this publication, only 1 woman has served as president for ABOMS (2011–2012) and for ACOMS (2018–2019); AAOMS has yet to elect a female president for its Board of Trustees.[16–18]

ADDRESSING RACIAL AND GENDER DIVERSITY IN MEDICINE AND DENTISTRY

The staggering statistics that demonstrate underrepresentation of minorities (ie, blacks and Hispanics) and women in the field of medicine, dentistry, and OMS call for an improvement in diversity within health care professionals in order to better serve the diverse American population and strive to resolve health disparities in the United States. This task can be addressed, in part, by

focusing on the recruitment of underrepresented students in high school and college, with continued mentorship throughout their education in professional school, residency, and/or fellowship, as junior health care professionals and faculty who are just beginning their careers and beyond.

Perhaps one of the most, if not the most, important aspects of recruitment, retention, and the development of health care professionals is that of mentorship, which has a positive impact on academic medicine and dentistry in clinical and research productivity, personal and career development, and advancement in higher academic ranks and governance boards. Although mentorship from senior faculty is crucial in the development of all health care professionals, underrepresented students and trainees relate most to mentors from the same or similar cultural or ethnic background. With the increase in mentorship for underrepresented minority (URM) students, residents, and faculty, an increase in

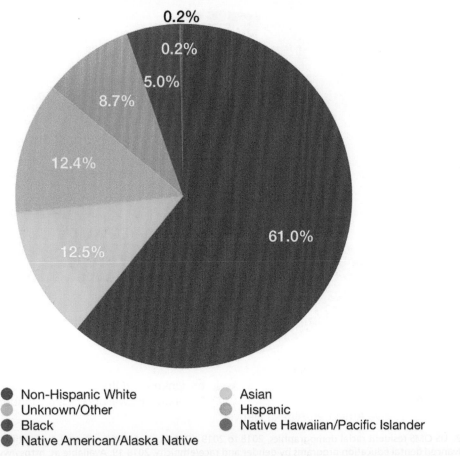

Fig. 8. US dental school faculty racial demographics, 2016 to 2017. (*Data from* American Dental Education Association. Full-time dental school faculty by gender, and race and ethnicity, 2016-17 academic year. Available at: https://www.adea.org/Fulltime_Dental_School_Faculty_by_Gender_and_Race_and_Ethnicity_2016-17_Academic_Year.pptx.)

recruitment, retention, and development of minority health care professionals in academic medicine, dentistry, and the health care workforce are likely to occur.

Funded by the W.K. Kellogg Foundation and led by 16 health, education, legal, and business leaders headed by former US Health and Human Services Secretary, Dr Louis W. Sullivan, the report of the Sullivan Commission on Diversity in the Healthcare Workforce was published in 2004 and aimed at identifying and understanding the barriers in achieving diversity in the health professions and finding solutions to these barriers.[24] Their conclusions and recommendations focus on equality in access to high-quality care for the entire US population, with diversity a key to excellence in health care, which can be achieved only by well-trained, qualified, and culturally competent health care professionals mirroring the diversity of the population they serve.[24] The report emphasizes providing public awareness campaigns to

encourage URMs to pursue a career in health care while health care professional schools financially support socioeconomically disadvantaged students and encourage the AAMC and American Dental Education Association to ensure a diverse student body with enhanced language and cultural competency, with emphasis on diversity being a core value in the health professions. This report also aimed at encouraging the increase in representation of minority faculty on major institutional committees, including governance boards and advisory councils, who often informally serve as mentors to aspiring underrepresented health care professionals.[24]

Racial and Gender Diversity in Medicine, Dentistry, and Oral and Maxillofacial Surgery

The Decision for Dentistry and Gateway to Dentistry programs at Rutgers University School of Dental Medicine for high school students and college

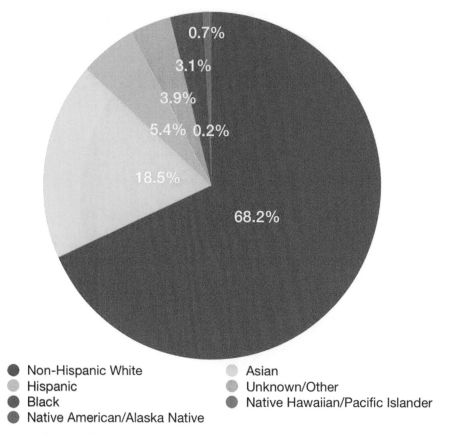

Fig. 9. US OMS resident racial demographics, 2018 to 2019. (*Data from* American Dental Association. Enrollment in advanced dental education programs by gender and race/ethnicity, 2018-19. Available at: https://www.ada.org/en/~/media/ADA/Science%20and%20Research/HPI/Files/SADV_2018-19.)

students, respectively, introduce URM students to a career in dentistry and its subspecialties. Although these programs are not tailored directly toward minority students, the high-school based program, Decision for Dentistry, enrolled more than 60% of students from URM groups.[25,26]

There also have been efforts to bridge the gender gap within medicine and dentistry, which strive to address the main contributors to this discrepancy directly, including the lack of appropriate female role models and mentorship to encourage the education and training of women, especially within the medical and dental subspecialties in which women are underrepresented.[27] In an effort to raise awareness and educate in order to alleviate this gender gap, the University of Michigan School of Dentistry and the Department of Oral and Maxillofacial Surgery hosted its first Women in Oral & Maxillofacial Surgery Leadership Symposium in 2018 to provide a platform for women and men to discuss opportunities and challenges faced by female surgeons and to promote leadership and career development along with networking for women in OMS.[28]

Similar interest groups in medicine exist, which also strive to enhance representation and experience for women, especially in academics. The Stanford University School of Medicine Provost's Advisory Committee on the Status of Women Faculty was created in 2001, where intensive access to influential faculty who served as role models and gender-directed mentorship led to successful career advancement, with the increase of women faculty to higher academic ranks, such as associate professorship and full professorship (87% and 75%, respectively).[27,29]

Finally, with positive mentorship, the development of URMs and women in health care professions and, more specifically, academic and organized medicine and dentistry, likely will lead to diversification of minorities and women in leadership positions and on governance boards. Diversification of health care professionals in organized medicine and dentistry will help alleviate health disparities as these governing bodies shape health care policies at the local and national levels.

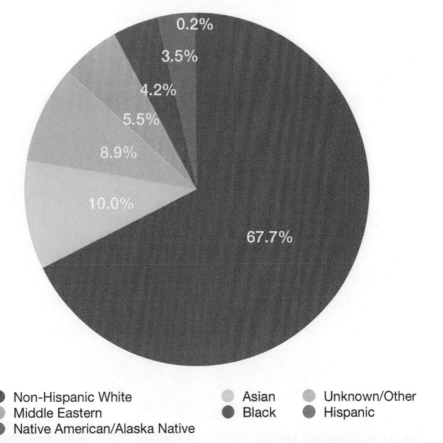

Fig. 10. US OMS full-time faculty racial demographics, 2019 to 2020. (*Data from* American Association of Oral and Maxillofacial Surgery. 2019-2020 Faculty members summary report. Personal communication.)

Cultural Competency in Medicine, Dentistry, and Oral and Maxillofacial Surgery

As medical and dental providers in the United States become a more diverse population of health care providers, their education and training also should reflect the diversifying patient population to aid in their ability to care for patients with diverse social and cultural backgrounds, values, beliefs, and linguistic needs. Studies have shown that health care providers who are from the same race or ethnicity of a particular region are more likely to serve in these communities. For example, dentists in Texas serve a higher percentage of black and low-income patients compared with white dentists, and racial or ethnic minority dentists are twice as likely as white dentists to accept new Medicaid patients.[30,31]

The existence of this disparity, however, often is a 2-way street, in that health disparities among minority patients in the United States is, to a certain extent, self-imposed, because many of these patients prefer to be cared for by health care providers of the same race or ethnicity.[32] Although there are no evidence-based data to suggest that racial or ethnic concordance between the provider and patient results in improved outcomes for the patient, lack of communication (eg, secondary to a language barrier), culture insensitivity, or lack of trust between racial or ethnic backgrounds can create a barrier to care and, thus, may bias a patient to obtain health care from a provider of the same race or ethnic group or to not receive care at all, which ultimately impedes the provision of acceptable health care.[33,34]

Cultural Competency Training in Medicine

In anticipation of a diversifying population, it is imperative that cultural competency training be incorporated into medical and dental education to train health care providers who are prepared to care for a diverse patient population. The Accreditation Council for Graduate Medical Education (ACGME) sets out an outline for medical residency and subspecialty program requirements and assesses programs for accreditation based on these guidelines. The ACGME mandates the fulfillment of 6 core competency domains by

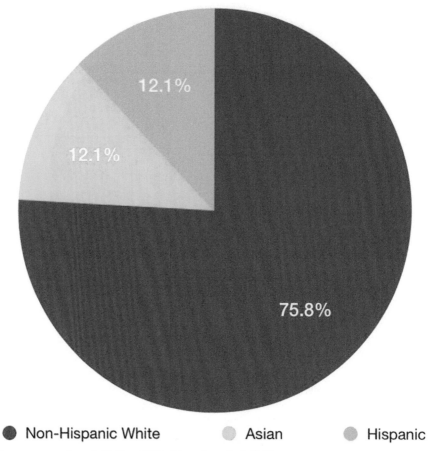

Fig. 11. OMS governance board, 2019 to 2020. (*Data from* Refs.[16–18])

postgraduate trainees during residency, which include practice-based learning and improvement, patient care and procedural skills, systems-based practice, medical knowledge, interpersonal and communication skills, and professionalism.[35] Although cultural competency is not explicitly defined as 1 of the 6 core competencies, it is relevant to 3 competencies, including patient care, interpersonal and communication skills, and professionalism.

There is, however, a paucity of data in the way in which cultural competency training is structured and measured for adequate competency, and there is wide variability without standardization in the specificity of cultural competency requirements among the 27 ACGME-accredited medical and surgical specialties.[36] Primary care specialties, identified by the World Health Organization as family medicine, internal medicine, obstetrics and gynecology, pediatrics, and psychiatry, were found to have more specific and concrete delineation of cultural competency training requirements in their curricula in comparison to

specialties, such as general surgery, plastic surgery, and urology, which were found to have less-specific cultural training requirements.[36] Although the higher emphasis on cultural competency training within primary care specialties likely is due to the role these providers play in patient care, with more-intensive direct patient interaction, the overall level of cultural competency training in postgraduate training remains highly variable, with few data on the acquisition of cultural competence for trainees.

Cultural Competency Training in Dentistry and Oral and Maxillofacial Surgery

Cultural competency training has been integrated into predoctoral dental education as per the accreditation standards of US dental schools, striving to train dentists who are "competent in managing a diverse patient population and have interpersonal and communication skills to function successfully in a multicultural work environment."[37] To achieve this competency, dental schools across the United States incorporate

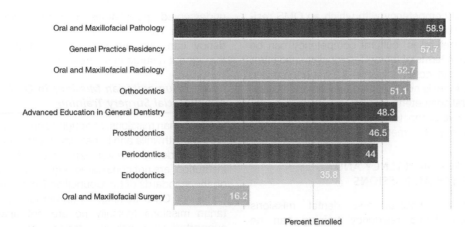

Fig. 12. Women enrolled in postgraduate dental residency, 2018 to 2019. (*Data from* American Dental Association. 2018-2019 Survey of advanced dental education. Available at: https://www.ada.org/~/media/ADA/Science%20and%20Research/HPI/Files/SADV_2018-19.xlsx?la=en; and Burke AB, Cheng KL, Han JT, et al. Is gender associated with success in oral and maxillofacial surgery? J Oral Maxillofac Surg 2019;77:240–6.)

patient and clinical experiences, such as rotations in underserved populations or through didactic courses.[38] Similar to cultural competency training in medicine, the incorporation of these types of experiences for dental students often lacks standardization among dental schools in their implementation and assessment of cultural competency, and few schools offer a dedicated, stand-alone course devoted to this topic.[38]

OMS residency programs are evaluated based on standards outlined in the *Benchmarks in Oral and Maxillofacial Surgery Education and Train*ing manual, developed by the AAOMS Committee on

Residency Education and Training and OMS Faculty Section Executive Committee, and reviewed by the AAOMS Board of Trustees. These benchmarks aid in the evaluation OMS residents during their training and are intended to increase the use of outcomes measurement in assessment in the OMS residency education process.[39] These benchmarks assess residents' abilities to treatment plan and manage patients with various diagnoses in addition to assessing their ability to effectively communicate with patients and families along with exhibiting ethical behavior and professionalism. There is, however, no specific assessment

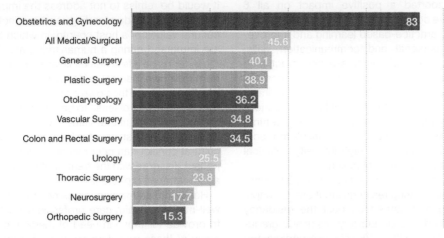

Fig. 13. Women enrolled in postgraduate surgical residency, 2017 to 2018. (*Data from* Murphy B. These medical specialties have the biggest gender imbalances. In: American Medical Association. 2019. Available at: https://www.ama-assn.org/residents-students/specialty-profiles/these-medical-specialties-have-biggest-gender-imbalances; and Lee JS, Ji YD, Kushner H, et al. Residency interview experiences in oral and maxillofacial surgery differ by gender and affect residency ranking. J Oral Maxillofac Surg 2019;77(11):2179–95.)

for cultural competency with which an OMS resident is evaluated.[39] Similar to that of the ACGME core competencies, cultural competency can be assessed in terms of the professionalism and interpersonal and communication skills benchmarks. Because there is no dedicated benchmark assessing cultural competency of OMS residents, it is difficult to assess the level of cultural competency based on objective measures.

CULTURAL COMPETENCY AND HUMANITARIAN MISSIONS

Humanitarian medical and dental missions completed during residency training can be considered a means of addressing and developing cultural competency. The availability of global health training opportunities provided to medical and dental residents often are sought out by potential applicants, and residency programs with established international opportunities favorably influence resident recruitment.[40] Although surgical trainees have participated in humanitarian missions for decades, in recent years, there has been a surge in trainees seeking international surgical experience to augment their training, and the long-term benefits for trainees participating in humanitarian missions are evident.[41,42] In a 10-year follow-up study evaluating plastic surgery resident experiences with Operation Smile, an international not-for-profit organization that specializes in the treatment of patients with cleft lip and palate, not only did surgical resident participants of Operation Smile report the development of their surgical skills during the mission but also a majority of participants reported a positive impact on all 6 ACGME core competencies: patient care, medical knowledge, practice-based learning and improvement, interpersonal and communication skills, professionalism, and systems-based practice.[42] Cultural competency is woven into these 6 ACGME competencies, to which surgical trainees reported improvement in their cultural awareness by becoming fully immersed in a diverse setting, that otherwise would have been difficult to reach, and participating in high-intensity clinical screening and operative planning.[42]

There are additional benefits to joining a humanitarian mission during residency that are, perhaps, long lasting and carried on past the residency training period. Plastic surgery residency graduates of the University of Virginia who participated in missions as residents were more likely to continue participating in future missions throughout their career compared with those who did not (60% vs 5.9%, respectively), demonstrating that the commitment to working with underserved populations cultivated during a short-term international experience during residency can translate into continued dedication throughout a surgeon's career.[42]

Role of Humanitarian Missions in Oral and Maxillofacial Surgery Training

Humanitarian missions, although generally considered a worthwhile and beneficial way to augment a OMS residency training experience at a home institution, are not considered requirements based on the standards of the Council on Dental Accreditation for OMS training.[43] Furthermore, humanitarian missions typically no are not financially supported by a resident's training program and must be funded either privately by the resident or through personally acquired scholarships. This financial burden often acts as a barrier to those who wish to become involved in humanitarian missions. There is, however, a growing interest and emphasis on the value of OMS trainees on a humanitarian missions not only to augment their surgical training within the field of OMS, such as cleft and craniofacial surgery, but also to develop the intangible patient-related skills that help trainees become well-rounded health care providers for a diversifying world. OMS trainees participating in humanitarian cleft missions reported that the participation in these missions developed not only cultural awareness and values of the host country but also their surgical skills.[43]

Role of Cultural Competency Training for Humanitarian Missions

It would be remiss to not address the importance of identifying, understanding, and respecting the cultural values of a host country in which trainees are immersed during a humanitarian mission and the differing beliefs in health, illness, and treatment from their own medical or dental training. Trainees must be aware of their own cultural values and beliefs in health and disease to be able to identify and understand the cultural values and beliefs of the people in the host country because potential for cultural conflict can occur when a provider and a patient disagree with the treatment recommended and treatment expected.

Humanitarian mission teams typically consist of well-meaning health care professionals who wish to provide for those in need of medical care, but many of these providers are not adequately prepared to treat patients with differing cultural beliefs in another country.[44] Currently, the World Health Organization provides guidelines for best practices health care; however, there is no international body overseeing short-term medical mission health care practices or its outcomes. Although much of this education in cultural competency typically occurs during the mission, professionals traveling with humanitarian mission groups, ideally, should be oriented with premission trip training that provides clinical and cultural training specific to that host country, which aids in educating the differences in values and beliefs in health and illness that exist among the host and providers' cultures. Due to the nature of timeline for these humanitarian missions, however, coordinating extensive premission trip training often is difficult secondary to time constraints and language barriers. Even a 2-hour, culturally sensitive educational program administered to medical professionals going on a short-term medical mission, however, demonstrated an improvement in their cultural competency, striving to ensure that standards of care to vulnerable populations are met.[44] These programs allow health care professionals to observe and understand a host community's beliefs and values, which, in turn, establish trust and adjust advice and actions while caring for these patients.[45]

SUMMARY

As the world becomes more diverse, it is imperative that the health care professional workforce is trained to care for the diversifying patient population, striving to improve health disparities in the United States and worldwide. This change can be possible only with active recruitment of URMs and women during their preprofessional school training and retention, with mentorship throughout their predoctoral and postgraduate training, and throughout their professional careers, with meaningful representation in medical and dental leadership positions and governance boards at the local and national levels. Improving the diversity within the health care professional workforce likely will aid in emphasizing the importance of cultural competency of health care professionals, with the development of programs aimed at cultural competency training and assessment, leading to a health care professional workforce ready to meet the needs and standards of the diversifying patient population in the United States and vulnerable patient populations abroad.

DISCLOSURE

The authors have nothing to disclose.

REFERENCES

1. Frieden TR. Centers for Disease Control and Prevention (CDC) health disparities and inequalities report: United States, 2013. MMWR Morb Mortal Wkly Rep 2013;62(Suppl):1–2. Available at: https://www.cdc.gov/mmwr/pdf/other/su6203.pdf. Accessed August 12, 2019.
2. US Department of Health and Human Services. Oral health in America: a report of the surgeon general—Executive summary. Rockville (MD): National Institute of Dental and Craniofacial Research; 2000. Available at: https://www.nidcr.nih.gov/sites/default/files/2017-10/hck1ocv.%40www.surgeon.fullrpt.pdf. Accessed August 12, 2019.
3. American College of Physicians. Racial and ethnic disparities in health care, updated. 2010. Available at: https://www.acponline.org/system/files/documents/advocacy/current_policy_papers/assets/racial_disparities.pdf. Accessed August 12, 2019.
4. Bach P, Pham HH, Schrag D, et al. Primary care physicians who treat blacks and whites. N Engl J Med 2004;351:575–84.
5. Reschovsky J, O'Malley AS. Do primary care physicians treating minority patients report problems delivering high-quality care? Health Aff 2008;27:w222–31.
6. Halbert CH, Armstrong K, Gandy OH, et al. Racial differences in trust in health care providers. Arch Intern Med 2006;166:896–901.
7. United States Census Bureau. US census bureau quick facts: United States. 2018. Available at: https://www.census.gov/quickfacts/fact/table/US/PST045218. Accessed August 12, 2019.
8. Association of American Medical Colleges. Diversity in the physician workforce: facts & figures 2014. Available at: http://wwwaamcdiversityfactsandfigures.org/section-ii-current-status-of-us-physician-workforce/indexhtml#fig1. Accessed August 12, 2019.
9. Association of American Medical Colleges. Total US medical school enrollmentby race/ethnicity (alone) and sex, 2015-2016 through 2019-2020. Available at: https://www.aamc.org/system/files/2019-11/2019_FACTS_Table_B-3.pdf. Accessed November 12, 2019.
10. Association of American Medical Colleges. US medical school faculty by sex and race/ethnicity. 2018. Available at: https://www.aamc.org/system/files/reports/1/18table8.pdf. Accessed November 12, 2019.
11. American Dental Association. Dentist workforce by race/ethnicity. 2016. Available at: https://www.ada.org/~/media/ADA/Science%20and%20Research/HPI/Files/HPIData_Profile_2016.xlsx?la=en. Accessed September 7, 2019.
12. American Dental Association. 2018-2019 Survey of dental education. Available at: https://www.ada.org/~/media/ADA/Science%20and%20Research/HPI/Files/SDE1_2018-19.xlsx?la=en. Accessed September 7, 2019.
13. American Dental Association. 2018-2019 Survey of advanced dental education. Available at: https://

www.ada.org/~/media/ADA/Science%20and%20Research/HPI/Files/SADV_2018-19.xlsx?la=en. Accessed September 7, 2019.

14. American Dental Education Association. Full-time dental school faculty by gender, and race and ethnicity, 2016-17 academic year. Available at: https://www.adea.org/Fulltime_Dental_School_Faculty_by_Gender_and_Race_and_Ethnicity_2016-17_Academic_Year.pptx. Accessed September 7, 2019.

15. American Dental Association. Enrollment in advanced dental education programs by gender and race/ethnicity, 2018-19. Available at: https://www.ada.org/en/~/media/ADA/Science%20and%20Research/HPI/Files/SADV_2018-19. Accessed September 7, 2019.

16. American Association of Oral and Maxillofacial Surgery. 2019-2020 AAOMS officers and trustees. Available at: https://www.aaoms.org/about/board-of-trustees. Accessed November 1, 2019.

17. American Board of Oral and Maxillofacial Surgery. 2019-2020 ABOMS board of directors. Available at: https://www.aboms.org/who-we-are/meet-board. Accessed October 29, 2019.

18. American College of Oral and Maxillofacial Surgery. 2019-2020 ACOMS board of regents. Available at: https://www.acoms.org/general/custom.asp?page=about. Accessed October 29, 2019.

19. Association of American Colleges. The 2019 Update: The complexities of physician supply and demand: Projections from 2017 to 2032. Available at: https://www.aamc.org/media/26541/download. Accessed September 21, 2019.

20. Association of American Colleges. Number of active residents, by type of medical school, GME specialty, and sex. Available at: https://www.aamc.org/data-reports/students-residents/interactive-data/table-b3-number-active-residents-type-medical-school-gme-specialty-and-sex. Accessed September 21, 2019.

21. Murphy B. These medical specialties have the biggest gender imbalances. American Medical Association; 2019. Available at: https://www.ama-assn.org/residents-students/specialty-profiles/these-medical-specialties-have-biggest-gender-imbalances. Accessed October 12, 2019.

22. Burke AB, Cheng KL, Han JT, et al. Is gender associated with success in oral and maxillofacial surgery? J Oral Maxillofac Surg 2019;77:240-6.

23. Lee JS, Ji YD, Kushner H, et al. Residency interview experiences in oral and maxillofacial surgery differ by gender and affect residency ranking. J Oral Maxillofac Surg 2019;77(11):2179-95.

24. The Sullivan Commission on Diversity in the Healthcare Workforce. Missing persons: Minorities in the health professions. 2004. Available at: https://depts.washington.edu/ccph/pdf_files/SullivanReport.pdf. Accessed September 21, 2019.

25. Rutgers University School of Dental Medicine. Gateway to dentistry. Available at: http://sdm.rutgers.edu/pipeline/gateway/gateway.htm. Accesses October 12, 2019.

26. Rutgers University School of Dental Medicine. Decision for dentistry. Available at: http://sdm.rutgers.edu/pipeline/decision/index.htm. Accessed October 12, 2019.

27. Gangwani P, Kolokythas A. Gender gap in leadership in academic medicine and dentistry: What are the barriers? What can be done to correct it? J Oral Maxillofac Surg 2019;77:1536-40.

28. University of Michigan School of Dentistry Oral and Maxillofacial Surgery/Hospital Dentistry. Women in Oral and Maxillofacial Surgery Symposium 2019. Available at: https://media.dent.umich.edu/sites/womss/. Accessed October 12, 2019.

29. Valantine HA, Grewal D, Ku MC, et al. The gender gap in academic medicine: comparing results from a multifaceted intervention for Stanford faculty to peer and national cohorts. Acad Med 2014;89(6):904-11.

30. Solomon ES, William CR, Sinkford JC. Practice location characteristics of black dentists in Texas. J Dent Educ 2001;65:571-4.

31. Okunseri C, Bajorunaite R, Abena A, et al. Racial/ethnic disparities in the acceptance of Medicaid patients in dental practices. J Public Health Dent 2008;68(3):149-53.

32. Saha S, Komaromy M, Koepsell TD, et al. Patient-physician racial concordance and the perceived quality and use of health care. Arch Intern Med 1999;159(9):997-1004.

33. Chen FM, Fryer GE, Phillips RL, et al. Patients' beliefs about racism, preferences for physician race, and satisfaction with care. Ann Fam Med 2005;3(2):138-43.

34. Mull JD. Cross cultural communication in the physician's office. West J Med 1993;159(5):609-13.

35. Accreditation Council for Graduate Medical Education. The milestones guidebook. 2016. Available at: https://www.acgme.org/Portals/0/MilestonesGuidebook.pdf?ver=2016-05-31-113245-103. Accessed October 12, 2019.

36. Ambrose AJH, Lin SY, Chun MBJ. Cultural competency training requirements in graduate medical education. J Grad Med Educ 2013;5(2):227-31.

37. Commission on Dental Accreditation. Accreditation standards for dental education programs. 2019. Available at: http://www.ada.org/~/media/CODA/Files/predoc.ashx. Accessed October 12, 2019.

38. Rowland ML, Bean CY, Casamassimo PS. A snapshot of cultural competency education in US dental schools. J Dent Educ 2006;70(9):982-90.

39. American Association of Oral and Maxillofacial Surgery. Benchmarks in oral and maxillofacial surgery

education and training. Available at: https://www. aaoms.org/docs/education_research/edu_training/ oms_benchmarks.pdf. Accessed October 12, 2019.

40. Bazemore AW, Henein M, Goldenhar LM, et al. The effect of offering international health training opportunities on family medicine residency recruiting. Fam Med 2007;39:255–60.

41. Campbell A, Sullivan M, Sherman R, et al. The medical mission and modern cultural competency training. J Am Coll Surg 2011;212:124–9.

42. Yao CA, Swanson J, McCullough M, et al. The medical mission and modern core competency training: A 10-year follow-up of resident experiences in global plastic surgery. Plast Reconstr Surg 2016;138: 531e–8e.

43. Aziz SR, Ziccardi VB, Chuang SK. Survey of residents who have participated in humanitarian medical missions. J Oral Maxillofac Surg 2012;70: e147–57.

44. Steinke MK, Riner ME, Shieh C. The impact of cultural competence education on short-term medical mission groups: A pilot study. J Transcult Nurs 2015 Sep;26(4):428–35.

45. Comninellis N. INMED international medicine & public health. 2nd edition. Kansas City (MO): Institute for International Medicine; 2012.

Travel/Tropical Medicine and Pandemic Considerations for the Global Surgeon

Christian Sandrock, MD, MPH, FCCP[a],*, Shahid R. Aziz, DMD, MD, FRCS(Ed)[b]

KEYWORDS

- Tropical medicine • Travel medicine • Preparation for global surgery • Pandemic • Public health
- Food-borne illness • Encephalitis • Tick-borne illness

KEY POINTS

- The traveling health care worker may become exposed to a wide range of tropical infectious diseases that occurs at the community and health care level.
- A pretravel visit and assessment is best performed before global surgical work.
- Universal precautions, including clean water preparations, food preparation, vaccinations, mosquito avoidance, and personal protective equipment use, will reduce risk.
- Some specific diseases, including malaria, arthropod-borne encephalitis, food-borne illness, rickettsia, and multidrug-resistant bacteria, are the most common infections encountered.
- In some cases, emerging pathogens, such as severe acute respiratory syndrome-coronavirus-1, will provide a particular risk for the departure, travel, and return home.

INTRODUCTION

International travel is often required for medical delivery to underserved communities. This travel requires preparation to prevent infectious diseases at the location of travel as well as diseases that can occur upon return.[1,2] Only a minority of illnesses will occur during travel, requiring a premature return to the home country.[2,3] Most of the illnesses will be minor and can be cared for locally. A recent study of 100,000 travelers (of all types) to the developing world stated that roughly 300 travelers will undergo hospitalization, 50 will be air evacuated, and 1 will die.[4,5] Surprisingly, most of the mortality and morbidity associated with travel remain cardiovascular disease and trauma sustained from motor vehicle accidents, not infectious diseases.[4,5] Recent literature suggests that infectious diseases account for less than 5% of

travel-associated mortality among travelers and health care workers (HCWs).[2,6] Mostly importantly, these infectious diseases are largely preventable, and a well-prepared HCW will largely have uneventful travel, allowing them to provide the maximal care to their patients. This article focuses on the basic generic preparation, prevention, and treatment of infectious diseases for the global HCW.

DIVERSITY OF TRAVEL AND DIFFICULTY OF PREPARATION

A traveler may be exposed to a wide range of infectious diseases during their global experiences.[6] These infections can come from the environment, community members, or most importantly, the local health care system. As such, the list of potential etiologic agents is very broad and hard to

a UC Davis School of Medicine, 4150 V street, Suite 3400, Sacramento, CA 95817, USA; b Rutgers School of Dental Medicine, 110 Bergen Street, Room B854, Newark, NJ 07103, USA
* Corresponding author.
E-mail address: cesandrock@ucdavis.edu

Oral Maxillofacial Surg Clin N Am 32 (2020) 407–425
https://doi.org/10.1016/j.coms.2020.05.001
1042-3699/20/© 2020 Elsevier Inc. All rights reserved.

differentiate and, most importantly, varies widely from location to location.[1,2] In general, travel-associated infections are acquired via enteral, respiratory, vector-borne, and/or sexual exposures. The most common travel-related infections can be categorized into gastrointestinal, febrile, and dermatologic illnesses.[3]

Thus, preparing for all diseases globally is an impossible task. Preparation must include reviewing the local epidemiology of the country visited. Even in these circumstances, local epidemiology can vary greatly given population migration, weather, vector growth, health care and public health infrastructure, and emerging pathogen presence. Thus, travel medicine must be tailored to the location. A few generic preparation actions can apply globally, and in many cases, a few diseases (eg, malaria, tuberculosis) can appear frequently across locations. In these cases, a broad preparation plan of education, vaccination, and basic disease preparation will provide care in most cases, with a few adjustments to complement the local epidemiology.

IMPORTANCE OF PREPARATION

At least 1 month before travel, an evaluation should be performed by a travel medicine or primary care physician[1] (**Box 1**). The pretravel evaluation should include the following:

- A review of all underlying medication conditions
- Pregnancy or potential pregnancy upon return home
- Allergy review and plans to assess allergies at location of travel (eg, medications)
- A review of the location for all vaccinations required
- A plan to take sufficient supplies of current medications because equivalent drugs may not be available in travel destinations
- An evacuation plan and review of travel insurance

Updates on needed prevention should be obtained via the Centers for Disease Control and Prevention (CDC; https://wwwnc.cdc.gov/travel). Specific country-based information and travel medicine guidance are found here. The evaluation should tailor the risks of the traveler, including comorbidities, to the location (see **Box 1**; **Box 2**, **Table 1**).[1–3] At the end of the session, a pretrip prevention plan should include vaccinations, medication supplies, water and food education, and an evacuation plan should illness occur (this will include obtaining evacuation insurance).

GENERAL PREPARATION
Water Safety

In most locations (not active war zone), bottled water or soft drinks should be present. If traveling to remote areas, clean water sources should be planned (see **Table 3**).[1,7] Travelers who have poor access to clean and safe water should purify water in the following ways[8] (**Table 2**):

- Boiling for 3 minutes followed by cooling to room temperature. Do not add ice to speed cooling.
- Adding 2 drops of 5% sodium hypochlorite (bleach) to a quart of water and letting sit for 30 minutes.
- Adding 5 drops of tincture of iodine per quart of water and letting sit for 30 minutes.
- Compact water filters with iodine impregnation can remove parasitic, bacterial, and viral pathogens.

Non–drinking Water Exposure

Swimming in fresh water can lead to multiple parasitic diseases. In areas of high schistosomiasis

---

Box 1
Basic pretravel appointment checklist

- Review all underlying medical conditions and comorbidities
- Review all travel locations
- Determine medication limitations at destination. If medication is unavailable, purchase supply of medications for travel
- Review medication and environmental allergies and take appropriate remedy (eg, epinephrine for nut/insect)
- Determine highest-risk activity on travel where infection is greatest (eg, altitude illness, fresh water exposure, personal travel safety and seatbelts)
- Review all vaccinations and determine those needed
- Review malaria risk and need and type of prophylaxis and discuss need for adherence
- Determine need for travel insurance
- Develop an evacuation plan in case of illness
- Plan home quarantine and return to work if returning from a high-risk area (eg, SARS-CoV-2 or Zika virus)
- Determine home-limited activities (eg, sexual activity, travel, avoidance of pregnancy) based on risk of transmission of disease (eg, Zika virus) at travel site

Box 2
General vaccines and prophylaxis required for global travel

Routine vaccinations

- Influenza
- Hepatitis B
- Hepatitis A
- Pneumococcal (If over age 65 years)
- Meningococcal (if age 14–25 years)
- Measles, mumps, rubella
- *Haemophilus influenzae* type b
- Polio
- Tetanus, diphtheria, pertussis
- Varicella
- Zoster if over age 50

Specialized vaccinations

- Typhoid
- Rabies
- Cholera (all areas of active disease)

(Asian, sub-Saharan Africa), fresh water exposure should be avoided, including short exposures such as rafting and boat rides.[9] Avoid walking barefoot or in loose-fitting footwear on beaches, on soil, or in water that may be contaminated with human or canine feces. Such exposure may lead to contact with *Strongyloides* larvae. Acquisition of the larvae can cause cutaneous larva migrans, hookworm, or strongyloidiasis.[2,9] Thus, limiting fresh water contact and wearing closed-toed shoes becomes essential in areas of high prevalence.

Food Safety

As with water safety, food safety is essential in regions where sanitation and personal hygiene are poor. Hands should always be washed before eating with appropriately treated water. Infections transmissible by contaminated food and water include traveler's diarrhea, parasitic infection, and hepatitis A and E.[10]

Raw foods rinsed with tap water should be avoided. Although chlorination may kill most viral and bacterial pathogens, the protozoal cysts of *Giardia lamblia* and *Entamoeba histolytica* and oocysts of *Cryptosporidium* survive and thus can be transmitted easily.[8,10] Basic advice for travelers should include choosing thoroughly cooked food served hot, fruits that the traveler peels just before eating, and pasteurized dairy products only.[8,10] Condiments on the table should be avoided because they can be contaminated. The old adage, "cook it, boil it, peel it, or forget it," is the best advice for food protection broadly.

Mosquito Protection

Global surgery often requires travel to regions with high rates of vector-borne diseases. The HCW should take action to reduce risk of bites from sandflies, ticks, and other mosquito species.[11–14] Basic measures should include the following:

- Avoiding outdoor exposure between dusk and dawn (peak *Anopheles* mosquitoes feed).
- Reducing the amount of exposed skin with clothing.
- Wearing clothing impregnated with insecticide (eg, pyrethrins). They are protective for about 3 washes or 3 weeks.
- Sleeping within bed nets treated with insecticide. These are protective for approximately 3 washes.

Table 1
Vaccines and prophylaxis specific to region of travel

Africa	Asia	South America	North America	Australia and Islands
• Yellow fever • Malaria prophylaxis chloroquine resistant (atrovaquone-proguanil, doxycycline, mefloquine, and tafenoquine)	• Japanese encephalitis • Malaria prophylaxis chloroquine resistant (atrovaquone-proguanil, doxycycline, mefloquine, and tafenoquine)	• Yellow fever • Malaria prophylaxis chloroquine susceptible		• Japanese encephalitis • Malaria prophylaxis chloroquine resistant (atrovaquone-proguanil, doxycycline, mefloquine, and tafenoquine)

Table 2
Basic preparations for environmental pathogen exposure

Water	Food	Insects	Other
• Boiling for 3 min • 2 drops of 5% sodium hypochlorite (bleach)/quart for 30 min • 5 drops of tincture of iodine/quart for 30 min • Compact water filters	• Cook it • Peel it • Avoid fresh fruits and vegetables • Hot and well-cooked foods from street vendors • No ice • Pasteurized dairy products only • No tap water for rinsing food	• Avoiding dusk and dawn • Reducing exposed skin with clothing • Insecticide-impregnated clothing (eg, pyrethrins) • Insecticide-impregnated bed nets • Well-screened or air-conditioned rooms • For exposed skin, wearing an insecticide, such as DEET, IR3535, picaridin, or OLE	• No open-toed shoes and fresh water • Avoid fresh water swimming • Seat belt use • Condom use for sexual activity • Avoid needle exposure if intravenous drug user

- Staying in well-screened or air-conditioned rooms.
- For exposed skin, wearing appropriate insecticide. This ideally is N,N-diethyl-m-toluamide (DEET), picaridin, ethyl butylacetylaminopropionate (IR3535), and oil of lemon eucalyptus (OLE).

Regarding insect repellent, DEET (30%–50%) is generally protective for at least 4 hours, although lower-percentage preparations provide a shorter duration of protection.[11] Picaridin, a synthetic repellant, has similar protection at 20% concentration when compared with DEET (35% concentration) for up to 8 hours. IR3535 (15% or higher) is protective for 8 hours, and OLE in is an effective repellant and can be used in children older than 3 years but has not been tested for efficacy or safety.[12–14]

Hand Hygiene and Personal Protective Equipment

As a global HCW, exposure to bodily fluids and contaminated fomites is common. As such, personal protective equipment (PPE) is paramount for the prevention of disease in both HCWs and their patients.[15–17] Health care systems can become a nidus for drug resistance and emerging infections. As such, the most effective preventive measures in the community include the following[15–19]:

- Performing hand hygiene frequently with an alcohol-based hand rub if hands are not visibly dirty or with soap and water if hands are dirty: 20-second vigorous wash is recommended before rinsing
- Wearing a surgical mask and face shield for contact and any procedures with bodily fluids (standard and contact precautions)
- When limited with mask, avoiding touching face, eyes, and mouth
- Practicing respiratory hygiene by coughing or sneezing into a bent elbow or tissue and then immediately discarding tissue and/or cleaning sleeve of shirt or skin at elbow with a disinfectant
- Masking all patients if they have respiratory symptoms. In resource-limited settings, using a cloth mask is appropriate

Precautions to be implemented by HCWs caring for patients include using PPE appropriately, specifically in how to put on, remove, and dispose of it. Taking these simple measures will protect the global HCW from developing a health care–associated infection while also protecting their patients in difficult resource-limited settings.

For maxillofacial surgery/head and neck surgery, appropriate PPE include the following[15–19]:

1. Surgical mask (level 3 or n95)
2. Eye protection
3. Hair covering
4. Surgical gown
5. Disposable gloves
6. Foot covering
7. Face shield

Antibiotic Resistance

Worldwide, the prevalence of multidrug-resistant bacteria (MDR) is rising rapidly.[20,21] Exposure to MDR occurs largely though food-borne or water contact. MDR strains have been identified in nontyphoidal *Salmonella*, *Shigella* spp, and *Vibrio cholerae*.[21] Gram-negative bacteria, such as *Klebsiella pneumoniae* and other *Enterobacteriales*, *Acinetobacter baumannii*, and *Pseudomonas aeruginosa*, are the most common bacteria found worldwide.[21–23] Treatment options for HCWs become limited for both their patients and themselves if they acquire disease in many developing countries. As a result, antibiotic treatment choices must be very tailored to the local epidemiology, and given the high rates of resistance, the use of PPE and sterile technique becomes essential in protecting both staff and patients.

Vaccination

The guidelines for recommended vaccinations for travel greatly vary based on the local epidemiology. However, despite this, several basic vaccinations, including yellow fever, meningococcus, typhoid, hepatitis A, hepatitis B, polio, and influenza are recommended.[24–26] **Box 2** and **Table 1** include the major vaccines that are recommended for travel to developing countries as well as some regional recommendations. However, as local epidemiology changes, up-to-date country-specific vaccine requirements can be found at the CDC (https://wwwnc.cdc.gov/travel).[24–26]

SPECIFIC COMMON DISEASES OF ALL TRAVEL FOR TRAVEL TO LOWER- AND MIDDLE-INCOME NATIONS
Malaria

Malaria is the most classic disease associated with travel.[2] Malaria is found worldwide and is common in most developing countries with varying prevalence and incidence. *Plasmodium falciparum* is the most common species to cause severe disease, with *P vivax* and *P malariae* rarely causing severe or respiratory-based symptoms.[27] Most cases can be mild and present both during travel and upon return.[28] All forms of malaria need treatment, except severe malaria require rapid treatment because of the potential for rapid decline and death within 24 hours of onset.[27] Malaria severity is often based on the parasite load, with less severe cases having 1% to 2% parasitemia and severe disease having 5% to 10% parasitemia (5% in low-incidence regions and 10% in high-incidence regions) with signs of organ damage.[29] The most common presentation is fever, headache, malaise, chest and joint pain, and weight loss. More severe cases progress with abdominal pain, jaundice, and splenomegaly and progress to the severe symptoms of altered consciousness with or without seizures, respiratory distress or acute respiratory distress syndrome (ARDS), hypotension and heart failure, metabolic acidosis, renal failure with hemoglobinuria ("blackwater fever"), hepatic failure, coagulopathy, severe anemia, and hypoglycemia.[27–29] Cerebral malaria with encephalopathy and seizures carries the worst prognosis.[27–29]

Artemisinin-based combination therapies for the treatment of uncomplicated malaria caused by the *P falciparum* parasite are the recommended mainstay.[30,31] By combining 2 active ingredients with different mechanisms of action, combination therapy is the most effective antimalarial medicine available today. Artemisinin and its derivatives must not be used as oral monotherapy, because this promotes the development of artemisinin resistance. In low-transmission areas, a single low dose of primaquine should be added to the antimalarial treatment in order to reduce transmission of the infection.[30,31] *P vivax* infections should be treated with an artemisinin-based combination therapies (ACT) or chloroquine in areas without chloroquine-resistant *P vivax*. Parenteral therapy is preferred for rapid treatment.[30,31] There are 2 major classes of drugs available by intravenous administration: the cinchona alkaloids (quinine and quinidine) and the artemisinin derivatives (artesunate, artemether, and artemotil).[30,31] Based on clinical trials, artesunate is superior for treatment of severe falciparum malaria when compared with quinine.[29–31] Additional support with blood transfusions can be considered in cases of altered consciousness, high-output heart failure, respiratory distress, and/or high-density parasitemia.[29–31] Exchange transfusion is additionally an option to reduce parasite load. Blood transfusion and exchange transfusion are largely supportive and have not been shown to reduce mortality.[29–31] Thus, they should not delay the onset of therapy with artesunate or quinine. In rare cases, nonfaciparum malaria can cause severe disease, and in these cases, treatment is identical with artesunate or quinidine.

Traveler's Diarrhea

Although bacterial pathogens predominate as the cause of traveler's diarrhea, viral and parasitic agents are also possible sources. Enteropathogenic *Escherichia coli*, *Salmonella* spp, *Campylobacter jejuni*, and *Shigella* spp constitute most of the worldwide causes of gastrointestinal disease.[32] Hepatitis A, rotavirus, and the parasites *E histolytica*, *Cryptosporidium parvum*, and *G lamblia* are the most common nonbacterial causes worldwide.[8,32] Up to 25% of individuals can have an infection with more than 1 organism.

Overall, the incidence of traveler's diarrhea is approximately 20% to 40% but varies greatly based on destination of travel, but the risk varies considerably based on destination of travel.[8,10] The highest-risk areas include South and Southeast Asia, Africa, South and Central America, and Mexico. Moderate-risk regions include Caribbean Islands, South Africa, Central and East Asia (including Russia and China), Eastern Europe, and the Middle East. Risk of traveler's diarrhea is highest during the first week of travel and then progressively decreases with time. High-risk activities include buying food from street vendors, traveling to visit friends and relatives, and staying in "all-inclusive" lodgings.[8,10]

The symptoms of traveler's diarrhea depend on the microbial cause.[8] The classic findings of enterotoxigenic *E coli* include malaise, anorexia, and abdominal cramps followed by the sudden onset of watery diarrhea.[8,10] Nausea and vomiting also may occur. A low-grade fever is variable. Most episodes of traveler's diarrhea occur between 4 and 14 days after arrival The illness is generally self-limited with symptoms lasting for approximately 1 to 5 days. The development of chronic gastrointestinal symptoms, and in particular irritable bowel syndrome, has been reported in a sizable minority of patients following traveler's diarrhea. Avoidance is the ideal therapy: only use known safe facilities (hotel, hospital, and so forth); never eat or drink from so-called street vendors. Once ill, acute management includes fluid replacement and rest.[32] Antimicrobial therapy shortens the disease duration to about 1 day, and antimotility agents may limit symptoms to a period of hours. Antibiotic treatment is reasonable for travelers with severe diarrhea, which is characterized by fever and blood, pus, or mucus in the stool, or for travelers with diarrhea that substantially interferes with the ability to work.[10,32] Antimicrobial choice depends on the region of travel but includes azithromycin, trimethoprim/sulfamethoxazole, and ciprofloxacin (or another fluoroquinolone). A restricted diet (eg, beginning with only clear liquids to match diarrheal losses during the acute phase of diarrhea) is often recommended.[10]

Encephalitis

Arthropod-borne encephalitis viruses represent a significant public health problem throughout most of the world and are found in all locales. They come from a wide range of families, such as Flaviviridae, Togaviridae, Bunyaviridae, and Reoviridae, and are highly adapted to particular reservoir hosts and region[33,34]. Spread occurs through an infected arthropod bite (usually mosquito or tick) and from animal to animal. The mosquito or tick becomes infected when feeding on the blood of the viremic animal, replicates in the mosquito or tick tissue, and ultimately infects the salivary glands. The mosquito or tick transmits the virus to a new host when it injects infective salivary fluid while taking a blood meal.

As a group, these viruses are found worldwide, but each specific virus has a regional presence. In North America, West Nile, St. Louis encephalitis, and La Crosse encephalitis viruses predominate.[35,36] Venezuelan equine encephalitis virus is of concern in Central and South America, whereas Japanese encephalitis virus affects persons living or traveling to parts of Asia.[33] Dengue is a rare cause of encephalitis throughout the tropical world.[37] **Table 3** outlines the major arthropod-borne viral diseases. Selected encephalitis infections are reviewed in later discussion.

DENGUE FEVER

Dengue viruses are spread through the *Aedes* species (*Aedes aegypti* or *Aedes albopictus*) mosquito. These mosquitoes are the same species of mosquitoes that also spread Zika, chikungunya, and other arthropod-borne viral encephalitis.[37–40] Dengue is common in more than 100 countries around the world with more than 400 million cases reported. Mild symptoms of dengue include a rash, nausea, aches, joint pain, and fever. Given the nonspecific findings, dengue can be confused with other illnesses that cause fever, aches and pains, or a rash. For mild disease, symptoms of dengue typically last 2 to 7 days.[37–40] Most people will recover after about a week. However, a minority of people progress to severe disease, especially in individuals who have had a prior infection with dengue. Symptoms of severe disease include the classic signs of hemorrhagic fever, including abdominal pain, jaundice, mucosal bleeding, and eventually hepatic, renal, and respiratory failure.[37] The diagnosis of dengue virus infection is established via serology or reverse transcription polymerase chain reaction (RT-PCR). Although mild

Arthropod-borne viral encephalitis

Disease	Viral Family	Vector	Geography	Symptoms	Treatment	Vaccine
Dengue	Flavivirdae	*Aedes* spp mosquito	Worldwide	Rash, nausea, aches, joint pain, and fever. Occasional progression to renal failure, hemorrhage	Supportive	No
Eastern equine encephalitis	Togavirdae	*Culiseta aedes, Coquillettidia,* and *Culex* spp mosquito	North and South America	Fever, headache, nausea, vomiting, minority with coma, stupor. Seizures and focal neurologic signs	Supportive	No
Western equine encephalitis	Togavirdae	*Culex* spp mosquito	North and South America	Headache, vomiting, stiff neck, backache, minority with coma	Supportive	No
Venezuelan equine encephalitis	Togavirdae	*Culex* spp mosquito	South and Central America	Sudden onset malaise, nausea, vomiting, headache, myalgia, nuchal rigidity, seizures, coma, and paralysis	Supportive	Equine vaccine
West Nile virus	Flavivirdae	*Culex* spp mosquito	Worldwide	Majority (80%) asymptomatic. Otherwise fever, headache, body aches, nausea, vomiting, skin rash, headache, neck stiffness, stupor, disorientation, coma, tremors, convulsions, muscle weakness, and paralysis	Supportive	Equine vaccine
Japanese encephalitis	Flavivirdae	*Culex* spp mosquito	Asia	20% asymptomatic. High fever, headache, neck stiffness, disorientation, coma, seizures, spastic paralysis	Supportive	Human and equine vaccine
Murry Valley encephalitis	Flavivirdae	*Culex annulirostris* mosquito	Australia, Papua New Guinea	Headache, fever, nausea and vomiting, anorexia and myalgias, malaise, irritability, mental confusion leading to cranial nerve palsies, tremor peripheral neuropathy, flaccid paralysis, seizures, and coma	Supportive	No

(continued on next page)

Table 3
(continued)

Disease	Viral Family	Vector	Geography	Symptoms	Treatment	Vaccine
Zika virus	Flavivirdae	*Ades* species mosquito	Worldwide, tropical	Low-grade fever, maculopapular pruritic rash, arthralgia conjunctivitis, congenital microcephaly, Guillain-Barré syndrome, myelitis, and meningoencephalitis	Supportive	No
Ross River Valley virus	Togavirdae	*Culex* spp mosquito	Australia, Papua New Guinea	Constitutional aches, fever (50%), rash, rheumatic manifestations, splenomegaly, hematuria, glomerulonephritis. Paresthesia, neuropathy, headache, neck stiffness, and photophobia, and encephalitis	Supportive	No
Chikungunya	Togavirdae	*Ades* species mosquito	Africa, Asia, South America	Fever, malaise. Polyarthralgia (bilateral and symmetric), macular or maculopapular rash	Supportive	No

disease is self-limiting, treatment of severe disease is largely supportive. Prevention of arthropod bites through covering and use of insecticides (DEET) is the primary way to avoid dengue.

EASTERN EQUINE ENCEPHALITIS

The eastern equine encephalitis (EEE) viruses (family Togaviridae, genus *Alphavirus*) consist of classic EEE virus found in North America and the Caribbean and Madariaga virus in South and Central America.[41–43] EEE virus is associated with severe clinical disease. In North America, wild birds and *Culiseta melanura*, a mosquito that is found in swampy moist areas, maintain the EEE virus. However, *C melanura* mosquitoes rarely bite humans; thus, some *Aedes*, *Coquillettidia*, and *Culex* species are responsible for transmission to humans. Although infections can occur throughout the year, peak incidence is in August and September in North America, and January and February in South America.[41] The incubation period is usually 4 to 10 days after the mosquito bite. The illness often begins with a prodrome lasting several days, with fever, headache, nausea, and vomiting.[42] A minority of people will progress to encephalitis, but, universally, disease is severe. Once neurologic symptoms begin, patients decline rapidly and progress to a coma or stupor. Seizures, and focal neurologic signs, including cranial nerve palsies, develop in approximately one-half of the patients. The diagnosis of EEE can be made by demonstration of immunoglobulin M (IgM) antibody by capture immunoassay of cerebrospinal fluid (CSF), a 4-fold increase in serum antibody titers against EEE virus, or isolation of virus from or demonstration of viral antigen or genomic sequences in tissue, blood, or CSF. Treatment is supportive. As with other arthropod-borne viruses, prevention focuses primarily on avoiding mosquito bites.[41–43]

WESTERN EQUINE ENCEPHALITIS

Western equine encephalitis (WEE) viruses (family Togaviridae, genus *Alphavirus*) are a complex of closely related viruses found in North and South America.[33] Spread is through *Culex* mosquitoes family, and thus, as flooding and increased standing water occur, regional outbreaks can occur. Incubation is about 7 days from a bite, followed by the onset of a headache, vomiting, stiff neck, and backache.[33] Restlessness, irritability, and seizures are common in children. Although rare in adults and older children, neurologic sequelae are relatively common in infants. The diagnosis of WEE can be made by demonstration of IgM antibody

by capture immunoassay of CSF, a 4-fold increase in serum antibody titers against WEE virus, or isolation of virus from or demonstration of viral antigen or genomic sequences in tissue, blood, or CSF. Treatment is supportive.[33]

WEST NILE VIRUS

West Nile virus (WNV) is a member of the *flavivirus* genus and belongs to the Japanese encephalitis antigenic complex of the family Flaviviridae.[35,44] WNV is commonly found in Africa, Europe, the Middle East, North America, and West Asia. WNV is maintained in nature in a cycle involving transmission between birds and mosquitoes. Mosquitoes of the genus *Culex* are generally considered the principal vectors of WNV. Humans, horses, and other mammals can be infected as dead-end hosts and are not part of the life cycle of the virus. The incubation period is usually 3 to 14 days. Most (80%) individuals infected with WNV are asymptomatic. For the minority who develop symptoms, fever, headache, tiredness, body aches, nausea, vomiting, skin rash (on the trunk of the body), and swollen lymph glands predominate.[35,44] Severe disease (also called neuroinvasive disease, such as West Nile encephalitis or meningitis or West Nile poliomyelitis) includes headache, high fever, neck stiffness, stupor, disorientation, coma, tremors, convulsions, muscle weakness, and paralysis. It is estimated that approximately 1 in 150 persons infected with the WNV will develop a more severe form of disease. Diagnosis is through antibody testing (IgM and IgG) in the serum with an appropriate 4-fold increase in titer or isolation of the virus in the CSF by RT-PCR.[35,44] Care is supportive. For those who develop neurologic disease, sequelae often persist. There is no vaccine at this time in humans.

ZIKA VIRUS

Zika is spread mostly by the bite of an infected *Aedes* species mosquito (*Ae aegypti and Ae albopictus*).[36,45,46] Outbreaks of Zika virus infection have occurred in Africa, Southeast Asia, the Pacific Islands, the Americas, and the Caribbean. In 2015 and 2016, a Zika virus outbreak occurred in the Americas, the Caribbean, and the Pacific. Besides infection through mosquito bites, documented infection has occurred through maternal-fetal transmission, sexual intercourse, organ transplantation, and handling of infected bodily fluids (eg, laboratory personnel).[36,45,46] Zika virus RNA has been detected in blood, urine, semen, saliva, female genital tract secretions, CSF, amniotic fluid, and breast milk.

Clinical manifestations of Zika virus infection occur in approximately 20% of patients and include acute onset of low-grade fever with maculopapular pruritic rash, arthralgia (notably small joints of hands and feet), or conjunctivitis (nonpurulent).[36,45,46] Infection has been associated with neurologic complications, including congenital microcephaly (in addition to other developmental problems among babies born to women infected during pregnancy), Guillain-Barré syndrome, myelitis, and meningoencephalitis. The diagnosis of Zika virus infection is definitively established by RT-PCR for virus RNA (in serum, urine, or whole blood) or virus serology. Treatment of Zika virus is supportive.[36,45,46]

Zika can be passed from a pregnant woman to her fetus. Infection during pregnancy can cause certain birth defects, and thus prevention, both with mosquito bites and with sexual transmission, is essential.[36,45,46] Pregnant women are recommended to prevent mosquito bites and sexual exposure to Zika during and after travel. If traveling without a male partner, one should wait 2 months after return before becoming pregnant. For male partners with a pregnant partner, condoms must be used, or one must abstain from sexual activity during pregnancy. Returning travelers should avoid being bitten for 2 to 3 months (viremic period) because this can establish disease elsewhere.[36,45,46]

CHIKUNGUNYA

Chikungunya virus is an arthropod-borne alphavirus transmitted by mosquitoes that predominately infects humans and nonhuman primates.[37,47–49] Chikungunya virus has spread from its origin in West Africa to Asia, Europe, islands in the Indian and Pacific Oceans, and the Americas. Infected travelers can import chikungunya virus into new areas, where local transmission can occur if competent mosquitoes are present. In Africa, chikungunya virus transmission occurs in cycles involving humans, *Aedes* and other mosquitoes, and animals (nonhuman primates and perhaps other animals).[37,47–49] Outside of Africa, major outbreaks are sustained by mosquito transmission among susceptible humans. Transmission via maternal-fetal route and blood products has been described, but unlike Zika and WNV, transmission through transplantation has not occurred. Incubation lasts from a period of 3 to 7 days followed by an acute infection with fever and malaise.[37,47–49] Polyarthralgia often begins 2 to 5 days after onset of fever and commonly involves multiple joints. The arthralgia is usually bilateral and symmetric, associated with morning stiffness,

and involves the distal more than proximal joints. Skin manifestations include macular or maculopapular rash. For most individuals, the duration of acute illness is usually 7 to 10 days; however, the inflammatory arthritis can persist for weeks, months, or years.[37,47–49] The chronic manifestations usually involve joints affected during the acute illness and can be relapsing or unremitting and incapacitating. Severe complications (including meningoencephalitis, cardiopulmonary decompensation, acute renal failure, and death) have been described with greater frequency among patients older than 65 years and those with underlying comorbidities. The diagnosis of chikungunya is established by detection of chikungunya viral RNA by RT-PCR or serology.[37,47–49] Testing for dengue, Zika, and Ross River Valley virus infection should also be considered because they present similarly. There is no known treatment of chikungunya other than supportive care.[37,47–49] Treatment of arthritis with nonsteroidal anti-inflammatories is recommended.

Tick-Borne Diseases

Rickettsia causes a wide range of human diseases across all continents. Rickettsial diseases are transmitted by ticks with a few exceptions: *Rickettsia prowazekii* is transmitted by a louse; rickettsialpox and scrub typhus are transmitted by mites; and *Rickettsia felis* is transmitted by cat fleas.[50]

The number of species of rickettsia is large, and important differences exist in the epidemiology, clinical features, and diagnostic methods.[50–53] However, the antimicrobial treatment is similar across all Rickettsia. **Table 4** outlines the major rickettsial diseases, and they range from African spotted fever to Rocky Mountain fever and scrub typhus.[50] The various clinical illnesses that are seen in association with the individual Rickettsia vary significantly in severity. Some, such as African tick fever, can be self-limiting with minimal symptoms. However, others, such as Rocky Mountain spotted fever, can progress rapidly if not treated and recognized. However, a few features do exist in common with all of them, including the following[54]:

- Rickettsial infections cause fever, headache, and intense myalgias.
- Rickettsial infections are arthropod borne; known or potential exposure to ticks or mites is an important clue to their early diagnosis.
- A rash or a localized eschar occurs in most patients.

After suspecting a rickettsial disease in a patient with a rash and fever, clinical diagnosis can be

Table 4
Most common Rickettsial diseases of travel

Disease	Agent	Vector	Geography	Symptoms	Treatment
Rocky Mountain spotted fever	*R rickettsii*	Dog tick (*Rhipicephalus sanguineus*, *Dermacentor*, *Amlyomma* spp)	North and South America	Fever, nausea, vomiting. Blanching erythematous macular rash evolving to petechiae. May have no rash (10%). Progresses to encephalitis, pulmonary edema, multiorgan failure	Doxycycline
Rickettsialpox	*R akari*	Mites (*Liponyssoides sanguineous*)	United States and Eastern Europe	Eschar at bite site, abrupt fever, chills, aches leading to papulovesicular rash	Doxycycline
Murine typhus	*R typhi*	Rat flea (*Xenopsylla cheopis*), cat flea (*Ctenocephalides felis*), and mouse flea (*Leptopsyllia segnis*)	Worldwide	Abrupt fever, aches, maculopapular rash at 7 d sparing palms and soles. May progress to neurologic, hepatic, cardiovascular, renal, and pulmonary failure	Doxycycline
Epidemic typhus	*R prowazekii*	Body louse (*Pediculosis humanus*)	Worldwide	Fever, headache, tachypnea, myalgias, rash, and arthralgias. Rash is maculopapular. Most patients with neurologic symptoms of coma, seizures, and cranial nerve deficits, Liver failure is rare	Doxycycline
Scrub typhus	*Orientia tsutsugamushi*	Trombiculid mites/chiggers (*Leptobrombidium* spp)	Asia Pacific Rim	Fever, headache, myalgias, maculopapular rash. May progress to myocarditis, pneumonitis, delirium, multiorgan failure	Doxycycline
African tick bite fever	*R africae*	Tick (*Amlyomma hebrasum*)	Rural Africa	Mild fever, headache, maculopapular rash (fine) over body, rate encephalitis, and myocarditis	Doxycycline

(continued on next page)

Table 4
(continued)

Disease	Agent	Vector	Geography	Symptoms	Treatment
Mediterranean spotted fever/ boutonneusse fever	*R conorii*	Dog tick (*R sanguineus*)	Sub-Saharan Africa, North Africa, Greece, India, Black Sea region	Eschar and black necrotic lesion at bite, papulovesicular rash similar to varicella. Rare neurologic complications	Doxycycline
Japanese spotted fever	*R japonica*	Tick (*Dermacentor, Haemaphysalis, Ixodes*)	Japan and Thailand	Eschar, abrupt fever, fine macular rash, thrombocytopenia	Doxycycline

achieved in 4 basic ways: serology, PCR detection of DNA in blood or tissue samples, immunologic detection in tissue samples, and isolation of the organism.[50–54] Often this is difficult in the field, and immediate treatment without a diagnosis is often recommended. The preferred treatment of choice is doxycycline, even for pregnant women and children, given the high rate of success. Alternatively, chloramphenicol can be used in adults. The route of administration will depend on the severity of disease, but most patients can be treated as outpatients with oral therapy.

Viral Hemorrhagic Fevers

Ebola/Marburg

The hemorrhagic fever viruses include wide number of geographically distributed viruses found worldwide, including Ebola and Marburg viruses, Rift Valley fever, Crimean Congo hemorrhagic fever, Lassa fever, yellow fever, and dengue fever.[55–57] Ebola and Marburg viruses are in the family Filoviridae. Although any of the many viral hemorrhagic fevers (VHFs) can cause severe disease in a traveler, Marburg and Ebola viruses serve as a classic template for VHFs and are largely discussed here.

Marburg virus has a single species, whereas Ebola has 4 different species that vary in virulence in humans.[56,58] Transmission appears to occur through contact with nonhuman primates and infected individuals.[59] Settings for transmission have occurred in vaccine workers handling primate products, nonhuman primate food consumption, nosocomial transmission, and laboratory worker exposure.[58] The use of VHF in bioterrorism has also been postulated, largely based on its high contagiousness in aerosolized primate models. The exact reservoir for the virus was initially thought to be with wild primates, but recently bats have been labeled as the reservoir, passing the infection onto nonhuman primates in the wild.[58]

The clinical manifestations of both Marburg and Ebola viruses are similar in presentation and pathophysiology, with mortality being the only major difference between them.[56] The initial incubation period after exposure to the virus is 5 to 7 days, with clinical disease beginning with the onset of fever, chills, malaise, severe headache, nausea, vomiting, diarrhea, and abdominal pain.[59] Disease onset is abrupt, and over the next few days, symptoms worsen to include prostration, stupor, and hypotension. Shortly thereafter, impaired coagulation occurs with increased conjunctival and soft tissue bleeding. In some cases, more massive hemorrhage can occur in the gastrointestinal and urinary tract, and in rare instances, alveolar hemorrhage can occur.[59] The onset of maculopapular rash on the arms and trunk also appears classic and may be a very distinctive sign.[56] Along with the bleeding and hypotension, multiorgan failure occurs, eventually leading to death. Reports of outbreaks and cases have largely occurred in developing countries where critical care resources are more limited.[58] Case fatality rates have reached 80% to 90% in the recent Marburg outbreak in Angola, but Ebola case fatality rates appear lower at 50%.[59]

The diagnosis of VHF becomes extremely important in order to initiate supportive care before the onset of shock, to alert and involve the public health department, and to institute infection control measures.[56,57,60] However, diagnosis is difficult outside of the endemic area. VHF should be suspected in cases of an exposed laboratory worker, of an acutely ill traveler from an endemic area (ie, central Africa), or in the presence of some classic clinical findings with increasing cases within the community suggesting a bioterrorist attack.[56] Outside of travel or laboratory exposure, the presence of a high fever, malaise and joint pain, conjunctival bleeding and bruising, confusion, and progression to shock and multiorgan failure should raise suspicion of a VHF, particularly if multiple cases are presenting in the community.[57] Laboratory diagnosis includes antigen testing by enzyme-linked immunosorbent assay or viral isolation by culture, but these tests are only currently performed by the CDC. Because no specific therapy is available, patient management includes supportive care, including a lung protective strategy with low-tidal volume ventilation if ARDS appears as part of the disease course. In a few cases in a Zaire outbreak in 1995, whole blood with IgG antibodies against Ebola may have improved outcome, although analysis showed these patients were likely to survive anyhow.

Although transmission appears to spread by droplet route, airborne precautions are recommended with respiratory protection with an N95 or PAPR and placement of the patient in a respiratory isolation room.[61] Equipment should be dedicated to that individual, and all higher-risk procedures should be done with adequate, full PPE. Any suspected case of VHF should immediately involve the public health officials and infection control department, because public health interventions and outbreak investigation will be paramount to reducing the spread of disease.[60] If exposure to an HCW occurs, there is no specific postexposure prophylaxis; infection control and occupational healthcare providers should be involved with potential quarantine measures for exposed individuals.[60]

Other Emerging Viral Pathogens

Coronaviruses

Coronaviruses are important human and animal pathogens and the source of approximately 30% of all respiratory tract infections worldwide. However, coronaviruses are a major source of emerging pathogens given their RNA genome, ability to adapt to multiple hosts, and the frequent contact between wildlife, domesticated animals, and humans. In 2003, a rapid progressive respiratory illness originating in China spread to multiple countries with more than 8000 cases and a case fatality ratio of almost 10%.[62] This disease was termed severe acute respiratory syndrome (SARS), and a novel coronavirus was determined to be the etiologic agent (severe acute respiratory syndrome-coronavirus-1 [SARS-CoV-1]). In September 2012, a case of novel coronavirus infection was reported involving a man in Saudi Arabia who was admitted to a hospital with pneumonia and acute kidney injury.[63] This case was followed by multiple clusters of infections in the Arabian Peninsula, and this outbreak was indeed related to a coronavirus (betacoronavirus), which is different but closely related to the other human betacoronaviruses (eg, SARS). In fact, this virus's lineage was closely related to bat coronaviruses. Within 12 months, more than 2400 confirmed cases of Middle East respiratory syndrome coronavirus (MERS-CoV) had spread to North Africa, Europe, Asia, and North America.[62,63] At the end of 2019, another acute respiratory syndrome was described in Wuhan, a city in the Hubei Province of China.[64,65] Likewise, this coronavirus is a betacoronavirus in the same subgenus but different class as the SARS virus. Based on the viral taxonomy, this virus was named severe acute respiratory syndrome-coronavirus-2 (SARS-CoV-2). This virus spread rapidly throughout China and with increasing cases worldwide, leading to an active pandemic. By May 2020, more than 1 million cases have been identified on 6 continents with more than 100,000 deaths.[64,65] Although cases of SARS-CoV-1 and MERS-CoV have all but disappeared, SARS-CoV-2 and subsequent disease from this virus (coronavirus disease 2019 [COVID-19]) are actively overwhelming hospitals and health care systems in North America, Asia, Europe, and the Middle East, thus altering the mobility and response of global HCWs.

Person-to-person spread of SARS-CoV-2 is thought to occur mainly via respiratory droplets, resembling the spread of influenza.[17,62,63] With droplet transmission, virus released in the respiratory secretions when a person with infection coughs, sneezes, or talks can infect via direct contact with the mucous membranes. The infection also occurs through the touch of an infected surface with subsequent touch to the eyes, nose, or mouth (fomite spread).[66] SARS-CoV-2 has been detected in nonrespiratory specimens, including stool, blood, and ocular secretions, but the role of these sites in transmission is unknown. Most importantly, spread through droplet mechanisms can be aerosolized when undergoing aerosol-generating procedures, such as intubation, bronchoscopy, tracheostomy, manipulation of the sinus and airway with surgery, and invasive and noninvasive mechanical ventilation.[61,65,67–69] This finding is important for any global HCW undergoing these procedures so that they have the appropriate PPE required for the given procedure to reduce transmission.

The incubation period for COVID-19 is thought to be within 14 days following exposure, with a median of 5.2 days.[17,64,65,69] COVID-19 ranges from mild to severe. Mild disease without pulmonary involvement occurs in approximately 80% of cases. Pneumonia appears to be the most frequent serious manifestation of infection, characterized primarily by fever, cough, dyspnea, and bilateral infiltrates on chest imaging.[64,69] Other findings, such as upper respiratory tract symptoms, myalgias, diarrhea, and smell or taste disorders, are also common. Severe disease (eg, with dyspnea, hypoxia, or >50% lung involvement on imaging within 24–48 hours) occurs in 14%.[64,69] More critical disease (eg, with respiratory failure, shock, or multiorgan dysfunction) was reported in 5%. The overall case fatality rate appears to be 1% to 2%, but a large number of minimal to asymptomatic carriers suggest that this case fatality rate may be lower. Comorbidities of cardiovascular disease, hypertension, diabetes, and immunosuppression appear to increase the likelihood of severe disease.[64,69] Male gender appears to be associated with a worse outcome along with various abnormal laboratory values: lymphopenia, elevated liver enzymes, lactate dehydrogenase, inflammatory markers (eg, C-reactive protein, ferritin, D-dimer [>1 µg/mL] and prothrombin time, troponin, and creatine phosphokinase). However, older age is perhaps most associated with increased mortality. In China, fatality rates were 8% among those aged 70 to 79 years and 15% among those 80 years or older.[64,69] There is a 2.3% case fatality rate among all other ages in contrast. It is also becoming apparent that some infected individuals become hypercoagulable, increasing the risk of embolic stroke or pulmonary embolism.[64,69]

Diagnosis is made by RT-PCR for viral RNA by nasal swab or respiratory sample. In areas of high prevalence, testing can help confirm the diagnosis in individuals with fever, cough, and other symptoms of COVID-19.[17,64,65,69] However, in areas of low prevalence, testing should be focused on individuals whom have had close contact with a known case of COVID-19 or have traveled from an area of high prevalence. Given the worldwide spread, targeted testing for individuals may not be indicated, and anyone with suggestive signs and symptoms should be tested.[17,64,65,69]

Infection control interventions to reduce transmission of COVID-19 include universal source control (eg, covering the nose and mouth to contain respiratory secretions and universal masking), early identification and isolation of patients with suspected disease (droplet or airborne precautions), the use of appropriate PPE when caring for patients with COVID-19, and environmental disinfection. Limiting transmission of SARS-CoV-2 is an essential component of care in patients with suspected or documented COVID-19. For traveling HCWs, an infrastructure of testing, isolation, and appropriate PPE is essential to decrease transmission to workers. In cases whereby inappropriate PPE is available, avoidance of work or travel is recommended.

Given the ongoing changes and evolving data around SARS-CoV-2 and COVID-19, global HCWs will need to follow some common guidelines to ensure safety for their equipment, patients, and team.[17,65,67,68,70] These guidelines include the following:

Pretrip preparations

- All members of a health care team travel should have a symptom screen before departure. If a fever is present along with cough, conjunctivitis, shortness of breath, or severe fatigue, a nasal swab for SARS-CoV-2 RNA by RT-PCR should be performed.
- Workers leaving from a high prevalence area (>10% infection) should have testing performed regardless of symptoms.
- Any worker with a positive test result should not travel. Return to travel or work should only be performed when symptom free for 72 hours or 2 successive negative tests 24 hours apart.
- PPE should include face shield, goggles, N95 or equivalent mask, surgical mask, gloves, and gowns. Confirm if your destination will have these, and if not, ensure that they are being secured with the team before travel.
- All PPE should be stored away from sunlight and in a low humidity area. Check all expiration dates on PPE before departure.

Arrival care

- All workers coming from a high area of prevalence who test negative before departure should self-quarantine for 14 days before working. This will ensure that disease is not spread to another area of lower prevalence, including patients.
- If symptoms consistent with COVID-19 develop on arrival or during work, begin isolation from workers and patients.
- If available, obtain a nasal swab for SARS-CoV-2 RNA by RT-PCR. Many developing countries will not have the resources to test. In this case, isolation until symptom free for greater than 72 hours and at least 1 week from the onset of symptoms will allow for a return to work. A mask should be worn for the next 7 days when working.
- For workers performing high-risk procedures (eg, intubation, surgical manipulation of the upper airway, bronchoscopy), screening of all patients before surgery should be performed. This should include symptoms screening, and any individual with symptoms consistent with COVID-19 should have surgery delayed.
- If possible, have local hospital perform screening by testing with RT-PCR. Because this is limited in developing countries, for patients who cannot receive testing but have no symptoms, appropriate PPE should be worn. This includes airborne precautions for any intubation or surgical procedure involving the airway and sinuses (PPE to include N95 mask, face shield, gown, and gloves).
- Patients with unknown test results should have a procedure performed in the operating room with a delay of more than 1 hour between cases to allow for more than 12 air cycles.
- If a local health care system has patients with active COVID-19, these patients should be cohorted and placed in droplet precautions (face shield, surgical mask, gown, gloves). If aerosol procedures are going to be performed, airborne precautions should be used during the procedure and for 1 hour after (roughly 12 air-cycle changes in room).
- HCW teams should monitor symptoms and wear a mask when unable to keep a greater than 3-m distance from each other.
- Intubations should be done in a rapid sequence manner. All patients should be orally intubated preferably with a skilled operator and video assisted if possible. Nasal intubations should be avoided. Bag valve mask use should be avoided, and the patient, once intubated, should be placed on the ventilator immediately without bag insufflation.

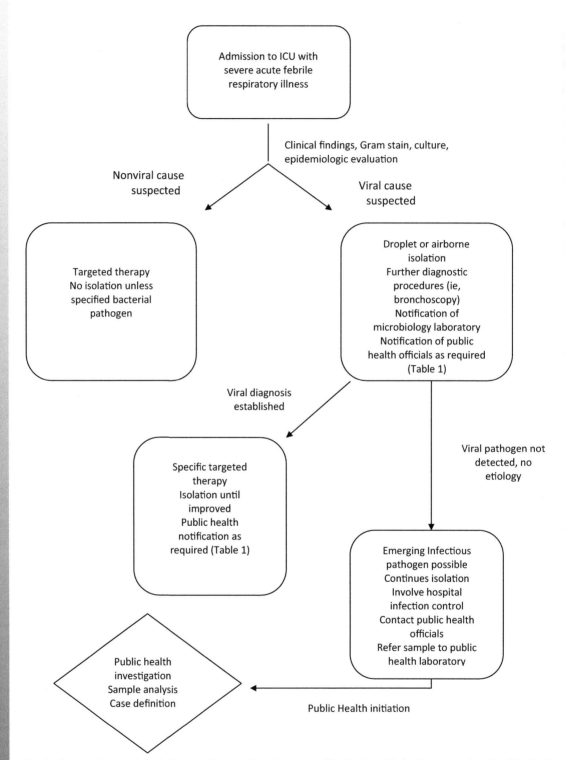

Fig. 1. Approach to early isolation, testing, and involvement of institutional infection control and public health in cases of acute febrile illness in a returning HCW. ICU, intensive care unit.

Posttrip preparations

- Upon return, all workers will have to quarantine for 14 days unless coming from a region with no cases.[6]
- Returning to work should be held off for 14 days.
- Avoiding family is recommended for 14 days as well, given travel from a high-prevalence region.

EMERGING PUBLIC HEALTH: WHEN YOU RETURN

If the returning traveler becomes febrile, if the cause of this fever is largely unknown, and if coming from areas of emerging pathogens, the evaluation and treatment can be difficult.[6,71] Although bacterial pathogens constitute most cases, the breadth of agents that can cause disease is enormous, with many having direct impacts on public health systems and the community.[61] Many of these cases require further epidemiologic and diagnostic testing, which can take time and resources in order to determine the larger impact of 1 ill traveler.[6] Often these patients will not be isolated and tested for these pathogens upon admission, and they will additionally undergo higher-risk aerosolizing procedures that will increase the likelihood for disease transmission.[61,70,71] Therefore, both HCWs and other patients are at risk for acquiring disease as experienced during the SARS-CoV-2 pandemic, the H1N1 pandemic, and other outbreaks of highly contagious disease.[60,61] Therefore, a standardized approach, with early isolation and testing of these cases, can reduce the likelihood of disease transmission of an emerging pathogen within the intensive care unit. **Fig. 1** outlines an approach to early isolation, testing, and involvement of institutional infection control and public health in cases of acute febrile illness in a returning HCW. Upon admission, the patient should undergo initial diagnostic testing as discussed earlier. If an etiologic agent is identified on initial screening and clinical findings (ie, gram-positive diplococci with a lobar pneumonia on x ray), targeted treatment is performed with appropriate isolation based on pathogen. However, if the agent is not easily identified in a patient with acute febrile illness and possibly pneumonia, patients should be placed in isolation, and further diagnostic testing should be performed based on epidemiologic risk. Isolation should most likely be droplet, but based on specific epidemiologic clues or high-risk procedures, airborne isolation may be instituted.[60,68]

Involvement of institutional infection control, microbiology, and public health should be started as early as possible.[68,70,71] Usually this is performed after the common agents have been eliminated and a suspicious high-risk pathogen is suspected.[60] Hospital-based infection control will assist in isolation and HCW protection, and the hospital-based microbiology laboratory should be notified of suspected pathogens, allowing for worker protection and targeted testing of samples.[68,70,71] Finally, public health involvement will allow a broader viral testing, including additional agents, subtyping, and resistance testing as well as rapid laboratory testing, epidemiologic investigation, case definition, and community prevention. Finally, higher-risk procedures should be limited in these cases. Appropriate PPE should be worn by HCWs at all time, and if worn properly, disease transmission is low risk.[68,70,71] Most cases during the SARS and the avian influenza epidemic appeared to have occurred when HCWs did not wear the appropriate PPE.

SUMMARY

The global surgeon may be exposed to a large number of pathogens through travel, including community exposure and health care contact. All global medical travel should begin with a pretravel visit whereby risk is assessed and all appropriate vaccinations and education are performed. Routine universal practices with clean water, food access, and insect avoidance will prevent most travel-related infections and complications. An understanding of the basic illness of malaria, traveler's diarrhea, arthropod-borne viral infections, tick-borne illnesses, and hemorrhagic fever will provide protection. Last, emerging pathogens that can cause a pandemic, such as SARS-CoV-2, should be understood to avoid HCW infection and spread in the workplace and when returning home.

DISCLOSURE

The authors have nothing to disclose.

REFERENCES

1. Freedman DO, Chen LH, Kozarsky PE. Medical considerations before international travel. N Engl J Med 2016;375(3):247–60.
2. Freedman DO, Chen LH, Kozarsky PE, et al. Spectrum of disease and relation to place of exposure among ill returned travelers. N Engl J Med 2006; 354(2):119–30.
3. Hill DR. The burden of illness in international travelers. N Engl J Med 2006;354(2):115–7.

4. Spira AM. Assessment of travellers who return home ill. Lancet 2003;361(9367):1459–69.

5. Spira AM. Preparing the traveller. Lancet 2003; 361(9366):1368–81.

6. Jimenez-Morillas F, Gil-Mosquera M, Garcia-Lamberechts EJ, et al. Fever in travellers returning from the tropics. Med Clin (Engl Ed) 2019;153(5):205–12.

7. Bacaner N, Stauffer B, Boulware DR, et al. Travel medicine considerations for North American immigrants visiting friends and relatives. JAMA 2004; 291(23):2856–64.

8. Steffen R, Hill DR, DuPont HL. Traveler's diarrhea: a clinical review. JAMA 2015;313(1):71–80.

9. Coltart CE, Chew A, Storrar N, et al. Schistosomiasis presenting in travellers: a 15 year observational study at the Hospital for Tropical Diseases, London. Trans R Soc Trop Med Hyg 2015;109(3): 214–20.

10. Shane AL, Mody RK, Crump JA, et al. 2017 Infectious Diseases Society of America Clinical Practice Guidelines for the Diagnosis and Management of Infectious Diarrhea. Clin Infect Dis 2017;65(12): e45–80.

11. Bohbot JD, Fu L, Le TC, et al. Multiple activities of insect repellents on odorant receptors in mosquitoes. Med Vet Entomol 2011;25(4):436–44.

12. Interlandi J. Insect repellents in the age of Zika. Our new tests identify what works and what doesn't against the bugs that can spread the virus and other serious diseases. Consum Rep 2016;81(7):40–3.

13. Katz TM, Miller JH, Hebert AA. Insect repellents: historical perspectives and new developments. J Am Acad Dermatol 2008;58(5):865–71.

14. Lupi E, Hatz C, Schlagenhauf P. The efficacy of repellents against Aedes, Anopheles, Culex and Ixodes spp.–a literature review. Travel Med Infect Dis 2013;11(6):374–411.

15. Anderson DJ, Podgorny K, Berrios-Torres SI, et al. Strategies to prevent surgical site infections in acute care hospitals: 2014 update. Infect Control Hosp Epidemiol 2014;35(6):605–27.

16. Ban KA, Minei JP, Laronga C, et al. American College of Surgeons and Surgical Infection Society: surgical site infection guidelines, 2016 update. J Am Coll Surg 2017;224(1):59–74.

17. Wax RS, Christian MD. Practical recommendations for critical care and anesthesiology teams caring for novel coronavirus (2019-nCoV) patients. Can J Anaesth 2020;67(5):568–76.

18. Liu Z, Dumville JC, Norman G, et al. Intraoperative interventions for preventing surgical site infection: an overview of Cochrane reviews. Cochrane Database Syst Rev 2018;(2):CD012653.

19. Munoz-Price LS, Bowdle A, Johnston BL, et al. Infection prevention in the operating room anesthesia work area. Infect Control Hosp Epidemiol 2018; 1–17.

20. Semret M, Haraoui LP. Antimicrobial resistance in the tropics. Infect Dis Clin North Am 2019;33(1): 231–45.

21. Hitch G, Fleming N. Antibiotic resistance in travellers' diarrhoeal disease, an external perspective. J Travel Med 2018;25(suppl_1):S27–37.

22. Ruppe E, Chappuis F. What and how should we tell travellers about antimicrobial resistance? J Travel Med 2017;24(2):1–2.

23. Nolte O. Antimicrobial resistance in the 21st century: a multifaceted challenge. Protein Pept Lett 2014; 21(4):330–5.

24. Rodrigues KMP, Moreira BM. Preventing diseases in round-the-world travelers: a contemporary challenge for travel medicine advice. Rev Soc Bras Med Trop 2018;51(2):125–32.

25. Sanford CA, Jong EC. Immunizations. Med Clin North Am 2016;100(2):247–59.

26. Freedman DO, Chen LH. Vaccines for international travel. Mayo Clin Proc 2019;94(11):2314–39.

27. Basu S, Sahi PK. Malaria: an update. Indian J Pediatr 2017;84(7):521–8.

28. Bouchaud O, Muhlberger N, Parola P, et al. Therapy of uncomplicated falciparum malaria in Europe: MALTHER–a prospective observational multicentre study. Malar J 2012;11:212.

29. Stanley J. Malaria. Emerg Med Clin North Am 1997; 15(1):113–55.

30. Griffith KS, Lewis LS, Mali S, et al. Treatment of malaria in the United States: a systematic review. JAMA 2007;297(20):2264–77.

31. White NJ. The treatment of malaria. N Engl J Med 1996;335(11):800–6.

32. Riddle MS, Connor BA, Beeching NJ, et al. Guidelines for the prevention and treatment of travelers' diarrhea: a graded expert panel report. J Travel Med 2017;24(suppl_1):S57–74.

33. Petersen LR, Hayes EB. West Nile virus in the Americas. Med Clin North Am 2008;92(6):1307–22, ix.

34. Kaiser R. Tick-Borne Encephalitis. Infect Dis Clin North Am 2008;22(3):561–75.

35. Petersen LR, Hayes EB. Zika virus. N Engl J Med 2016;374(16):1552–63.

36. Calisher CH. Medically important arboviruses of the United States and Canada. Clin Microbiol Rev 1994; 7(1):89–116.

37. Nicoletti L, Ciccozzi M, Marchi A, et al. Chikungunya and dengue viruses in travelers. Emerg Infect Dis 2008;14(1):177–8.

38. Guzman MG, Harris E. Dengue. Lancet 2015; 385(9966):453–65.

39. Kularatne SA. Dengue fever. BMJ 2015;351:h4661.

40. Simmons CP, Farrar JJ, Nguyen vV, et al. Dengue. N Engl J Med 2012;366(15):1423–32.

41. Carrera JP, Forrester N, Wang E, et al. Eastern equine encephalitis in Latin America. N Engl J Med 2013;369(8):732–44.

42. Deresiewicz RL, Thaler SJ, Hsu L, et al. Clinical and neuroradiographic manifestations of eastern equine encephalitis. N Engl J Med 1997;336(26):1867–74.

43. Wendell LC, Potter NS, Roth JL, et al. Successful management of severe neuroinvasive eastern equine encephalitis. Neurocrit Care 2013;19(1):111–5.

44. Petersen LR, Brault AC, Nasci RS. West Nile virus: review of the literature. JAMA 2013;310(3):308–15.

45. Baud D, Gubler DJ, Schaub B, et al. An update on Zika virus infection. Lancet 2017;390(10107):2099–109.

46. Musso D, Gubler DJ. Zika virus. Clin Microbiol Rev 2016;29(3):487–524.

47. Hochedez P, et al. Chikungunya infection in travelers. Emerg Infect Dis 2006;12(10):1565–7.

48. Staples JE, Breiman RF, Powers AM. Chikungunya fever: an epidemiological review of a re-emerging infectious disease. Clin Infect Dis 2009;49(6):942–8.

49. Weaver SC, Lecuit M. Chikungunya virus and the global spread of a mosquito-borne disease. N Engl J Med 2015;372(13):1231–9.

50. Walker DH. Rickettsiae and rickettsial infections: the current state of knowledge. Clin Infect Dis 2007;45(Suppl 1):S39–44.

51. Chapman AS, Bakken JS, Folk SM, et al. Diagnosis and management of tickborne rickettsial diseases: Rocky Mountain spotted fever, ehrlichioses, and anaplasmosis–United States: a practical guide for physicians and other health-care and public health professionals. MMWR Recomm Rep 2006;55(RR-4):1–27.

52. Jensenius M, Fournier PE, Raoult D. Rickettsioses and the international traveler. Clin Infect Dis 2004;39(10):1493–9.

53. Parola P, Paddock CD, Socolovschi C, et al. Update on tick-borne rickettsioses around the world: a geographic approach. Clin Microbiol Rev 2013;26(4):657–702.

54. Biggs HM, Behravesh CB, Bradley KK, et al. Diagnosis and management of tickborne rickettsial diseases: Rocky Mountain spotted fever and other spotted fever group rickettsioses, ehrlichioses, and anaplasmosis–United States. MMWR Recomm Rep 2016;65(2):1–44.

55. Iannetta M, Di Caro A, Nicastri E, et al. Viral hemorrhagic fevers other than Ebola and Lassa. Infect Dis Clin North Am 2019;33(4):977–1002.

56. Nicastri E, Kobinger G, Vairo F, et al. Ebola virus disease: epidemiology, clinical features, management, and prevention. Infect Dis Clin North Am 2019;33(4):953–76.

57. Asogun DA, Gunther S, Akpede GO, et al. Lassa fever: epidemiology, clinical features, diagnosis, management and prevention. Infect Dis Clin North Am 2019;33(4):933–51.

58. Oppenheim B, Lidow N, Ayscue P, et al. Knowledge and beliefs about Ebola virus in a conflict-affected area: early evidence from the North Kivu outbreak. J Glob Health 2019;9(2):020311.

59. To KK, Chan JF, Tsang AK, et al. Ebola virus disease: a highly fatal infectious disease reemerging in West Africa. Microbes Infect 2015;17(2):84–97.

60. Maves RC, Jamros CM, Smith AG. Intensive care unit preparedness during pandemics and other biological threats. Crit Care Clin 2019;35(4):609–18.

61. Sandrock C, Stollenwerk N. Acute febrile respiratory illness in the ICU: reducing disease transmission. Chest 2008;133(5):1221–31.

62. Christian MD, Poutanen SM, Loutfy MR, et al. Severe acute respiratory syndrome. Clin Infect Dis 2004;38(10):1420–7.

63. Arabi YM, Balkhy HH, Hayden FG, et al. Middle East respiratory syndrome. N Engl J Med 2017;376(6):584–94.

64. Guan WJ, Ni ZY, Hu Y, et al. Clinical characteristics of coronavirus disease 2019 in China. N Engl J Med 2020.

65. Zhu N, Zhang D, Wang W, et al. A novel coronavirus from patients with pneumonia in China, 2019. N Engl J Med 2020;382(8):727–33.

66. Wang W, Xu Y, Gao R, et al. Detection of SARS-CoV-2 in different types of clinical specimens. JAMA 2020. [Epub ahead of print].

67. Otter JA, et al. Transmission of SARS and MERS coronaviruses and influenza virus in healthcare settings: the possible role of dry surface contamination. J Hosp Infect 2016;92(3):235–50.

68. Sandrock CE. Severe febrile respiratory illnesses as a cause of mass critical care. Respir Care 2008;53(1):40–53 [discussion: 53–7].

69. Zhou F, Yu T, Du R, et al. Clinical course and risk factors for mortality of adult inpatients with COVID-19 in Wuhan, China: a retrospective cohort study. Lancet 2020;395(10229):1054–62.

70. Sandrock CE. Care of the critically ill and injured during pandemics and disasters: groundbreaking results from the Task Force on Mass Critical Care. Chest 2014;146(4):881–3.

71. Sanford CA, Fung C. Illness in the returned international traveler. Med Clin North Am 2016;100(2):393–409.

Global Anesthesia in Oral and Maxillofacial Surgery

Evonne Greenidge, MD[a,b], Michael Krieves, MD[a,c,*], Rene Solorzano, CAT[a,d,1]

KEYWORDS

- Low-resource environment • Global health • Medical missions • Cleft and craniofacial missions
- Pediatric anesthesia • General anesthesia

KEY POINTS

- Volunteer medical missions require careful planning and coordination between surgical and anesthesia teams, as well as the host medical institution.
- All equipment and supplies should be well thought out, because these items may be difficult to source in the host country.
- Anesthesia and perioperative nursing personnel should be comfortable with the care of pediatric patients and management of cleft lip and palate surgical patients.

INTRODUCTION

Perioperative anesthetic care for patients undergoing oral and maxillofacial surgical procedures can vary depending on the type of surgery and airway management involved. When considering the procedures to undertake during a surgical mission to low-income or middle-income countries (LMICs), anesthesia providers and surgeons should carefully consider the following factors: the patient's medical history; availability of equipment and supplies; backup resources, such as blood products; and the mechanism to provide postoperative care. For example, a patient with uncontrolled medical problems such as hypertension or chronic obstructive pulmonary disease should not be considered if appropriate postoperative care is not available in the hospital. In addition, procedures with the potential for significant blood loss that may require a transfusion should be avoided in a facility without a blood bank or the means to type or screen a blood sample.

Oral and maxillofacial surgery (OMFS) in an LMIC can involve multiple procedures, including repair for craniofacial deformities, vascular malformations, and facial masses. When providing anesthesia care, the goal should always be the safety of the patient.[1] The challenge for anesthesia providers is maintaining the standard of care in an environment with limited resources.[2] It is important to remember that, when deciding whether a procedure should be done, surgeons should consider whether it would be done in their home countries. In most cases, the proposed procedures are done for elective treatment of a congenital or acquired condition[1] and a procedure should not be done if it represents an increased risk to the patient in the perioperative period.

Repair of cleft lip and cleft palate represents most procedures done for craniofacial deformities[3] by oral and maxillofacial, plastic, or otolaryngology surgeons during surgical missions to an LMIC. Most procedures are performed in pediatric patients but adults do present for surgical correction or revision surgery. The anesthesia considerations for repair of orofacial clefts in pediatric patients are addressed primarily but information in this article is applicable to other procedures performed less commonly on pediatric and adult populations.

[a] Smile Bangladesh; [b] Private Practice, Washington, DC, USA; [c] Private Practice, Grand Junction, CO, USA; [d] Department of Anesthesiology, Columbia University Irving Medical Center, New York, NY, USA
[1] 2099 S Broadway, Grand Junction, CO 81507
* Corresponding author. 2099 S Broadway, Grand Junction, CO 81507.
E-mail address: Mkrieves@gmail.com

Oral Maxillofacial Surg Clin N Am 32 (2020) 427–436
https://doi.org/10.1016/j.coms.2020.04.004
1042-3699/20/© 2020 Elsevier Inc. All rights reserved.

CLEFT LIP AND PALATE REPAIR

The facial deformities, cleft lip and cleft palate, represent the most common craniofacial anomalies for elective surgical repair in infants and children. The defect can occur in isolation or together (ie, cleft lip only, cleft lip with cleft palate, or cleft palate only). These defects do occur in healthy patients but may occur with some associations significant for anesthesia care, including the potential for difficult airway management (**Box 1**).[4] Available data show that the incidence of cleft lip with or without cleft palate is 10.63 per 10,000 live births in the United States and show some ethnic variation, with the highest incidence in Native Americans, 3.6 in 1000 live births.[5] The incidence of cleft palate is 6.35 per 10,000 live births.[5]

The surgical correction of cleft lip (cheiloplasty) is a short procedure under general or local anesthesia. The repair is usually done within the first few months of life and can even occur in the neonatal period.[6] In contrast, cleft palate repair (palatoplasty) is usually completed before speech development, by age 2 years, usually at approximately 9 months of age.

The number of cleft lip and cleft palate repair procedures performed in an LMIC by visiting surgical teams is difficult to estimate. However, 1 study noted that there were approximately 3000 patients in a 4-year period from 2007 to 2010 ranging in age from 1 month to 64 years old at 1 hospital in India.[7] That number extrapolates to thousands of procedures performed annually throughout the world by hundreds of visiting surgical teams. Limited data are published about the surgical or anesthetic care during such procedures, but it is clear that visiting teams continue to make an impact even without providing details about their work.

The anesthetic care of patients for cleft repair can range from local anesthesia with an infraorbital block to general anesthesia with mechanical ventilation. The planning, equipment, and supplies needed to provide a safe anesthetic are discussed further later, in addition to the considerations for selecting patients and providing adequate follow-up.

PLANNING AND ORGANIZATION

The planning for an overseas surgical trip should start with enough time to adequately make a successful mission. This process may take up to a year for a new location within a limited-resource setting.

Goals

It is important to assess the goals for the trip in order to plan for all possible scenarios that may arise. When the team's primary objective is direct patient care, as opposed to education and training of local hospital staff, the need for local hospital personnel and equipment is more prevalent. For example, cleft palate repair on pediatric patients would require oral RAE (Ring, Adair, and Elwyn) endotracheal tubes, which may not be easily available in some countries. Similarly, the need for adequate monitoring, blood products, and postoperative care for complex oral surgery procedures may not be appropriate in some settings.

Personnel

After deciding on the anesthesia team leader, preferably the person with the most surgical mission experience,[1] the composition of the additional anesthesia staff should be determined. Planning for the anticipated age range for patients and number of procedures dictates the other members of the anesthesia team. For trips that will involve pediatric patients, having a board-certified pediatric anesthesiologist is advisable.[7] No one should be operating outside of their scope of practice or performing procedures that they are not authorized to perform in their home countries. In deciding whether to include trainees on the team, the appropriate level of supervision must be provided. It is advisable to include an anesthesia provider to cover the postanesthesia care unit, serve as a float for breaks and starting procedures, and to fill in if any unexpected illnesses or last-minute cancellations should arise. The addition of an anesthesia technologist or technician to the team can be extremely beneficial to address monitoring and access to equipment.

Box 1
Syndromes associated with cleft lip and/or palate

Deletion 9p syndrome

EEC (ectrodactyly, ectodermal dysplasia, and cleft lip and palate) syndrome

Ellis–van Creveld syndrome

Goldenhar syndrome

Median cleft face syndrome

Nager syndrome

Oral-facial-digital syndrome

Patau (trisomy 13) syndrome

Pierre Robin sequence

Stickler syndrome

Treacher Collins syndrome

Facilities

There should be a preliminary site visit before deciding on the location for the surgical trip.[1,8] At that time, facilities and support services should be assessed for the planned mission and pictures should be taken. The site visitor should assess the operating suite, including the number of tables, rooms, recovery areas, laboratories, radiology services, blood banks, and pharmaceutical services. The hospital should have a reliable source of electricity, oxygen cylinders, and water for the proposed surgical procedures.[1] The need for sterilization of instruments and safe storage of supplies and equipment used during the trip should also be considered. The availability of the laboratory to process preoperative or urgent laboratory specimens,[1] radiology for radiographs preoperatively or in an emergency, cardiology for electrocardiogram and echocardiogram evaluation, and the pharmacy for any medications for the trip should be assessed. In addition, the presence of a local pharmacy can serve as a reliable source for some medications.[1] The operating suite should be able to support the number of planned surgical procedures. The proximity of the recovery area and patient ward should also be considered in the event of any postoperative events.

Anesthesia Machines

The anesthesia machines available in the hospital may be unfamiliar to the providers and lack the safety mechanisms common in their home countries. Often the provider needs to adjust the anesthesia machine that is available to function for the planned procedures. The types of machines available include variable bypass, flow-over vaporizer, and draw-over vaporizer (**Fig. 1**).[1] The provider should be able to understand the functioning of the various types of anesthesia machines encountered if not importing anesthesia machines (Boyles, pneumatic, draw-over, Glostavent, or electronic machine) (**Box 2**).

If planning to use an electronic anesthesia machine, the provider should consider the availability of a reliable source of electricity. As an alternative, Khambatta and colleagues[2] described a safe, low-technology machine that only requires an oxygen tank, tubing, a vaporizer with connector, portable carbon dioxide absorber, and a breathing circuit. Unlike the machines discussed earlier, this system does not require electricity and can be easily transported compared with other machines. Scavenging of anesthetic agents is usually accomplished by using additional circuits configured to ventilate to the outside. The provider should be mindful of placement of the exhausted agents

and position the scavenging away from patients or other persons.

A reliable supply of oxygen cylinders with regulators and flow meters is necessary, preferably large H cylinders. Compressed air and nitrous oxide cylinders may be more difficult to source depending on location.

Monitors

The provider should plan for monitoring of patients in the operating room and the recovery room. The monitors available at the hospital may be partially or fully functional, so anticipate the need for supplemental equipment. In particular, a manual blood pressure cuff and portable pulse oximeter are extremely useful if no functional monitors are available or electricity is unreliable. Similarly, a precordial stethoscope also provides an assessment of the patient if monitors are unavailable. The American Society of Anesthesiologists (ASA) standards for monitoring are shown in **Box 3**.[9] In extenuating circumstances, some of the requirements can be waived or modified, but the reasons must be included in the patient's medical record. These standards represent those in the developed world but may not be available because of equipment availability in a limited-resource setting. Anesthetists should maintain a level of vigilance when outside their home countries when the required safety measures are not in place. For example, machines may make it possible to deliver 100% nitrous oxide to a patient. There also may be no low-oxygen alarms, so the anesthesiologist must regularly check the supply available from the cylinders.

Anesthesia Supplies

The availability of supplies should be assessed in the initial planning process to address the proper transport or purchase of supplies. This assessment avoids any delays with shipping, customs, and backorders. Practitioners may reuse appropriately sterilized disposable items if it is the normal practice of the home country.[1] A list with suggested supplies is shown in **Box 4**.

Medications

The medications, including anesthetic agents, intravenous (IV) fluids, and antibiotics, needed depend on the type of procedures planned. Total IV anesthesia with propofol, dexmedetomidine, and/or ketamine is an alternative if a functioning anesthesia machine is not available. There should be medications available for resuscitation in case of an emergency. A suggested list of medications is shown in **Box 5**.

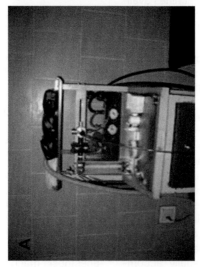
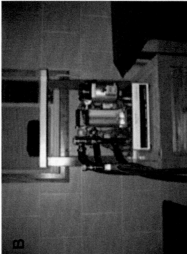
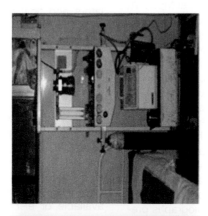

Fig. 1. (A) Goldman vaporizer. (B) Halothane variable bypass vaporizer. (C) Anesthesia machine.

Box 2
Anesthesia equipment

Anesthesia machine

Anesthesia vaporizers

Monitors

Anesthesia circuits: child and adult

Defibrillator

Suction

PATIENT SELECTION

The screening of potential patients should be done with the oral surgery and anesthesia teams. Ideally the local medical personnel complete the initial screening process, including history and physical, before the arrival of the surgical team. By completing the initial screening process, those suitable for surgery would have laboratory results, echocardiogram, and radiographs available on arrival of the surgical team. This system greatly facilitates the screening process, which sometimes involves hundreds of potential patients. Complexity of surgery, postoperative care needed, and advanced disease process should be considered when selecting patients.[1]

Each patient considered a surgical candidate should undergo a preoperative physical examination, including airway assessment, heart and lung examination, and determination of ASA physical status classification. Patients should be examined before the procedure for overall appearance,

---

Box 3
American Society of Anesthesiologists standards for monitoring

Qualified anesthesia personnel

Pulse oximetry

Capnography

Electrocardiogram (ECG)

Blood pressure at least every 5 minutes

Heart rate

Temperature

Disconnect alarm if using mechanical ventilation

Data from American Society of Anesthesiologists. Standards for basic anesthetic monitoring. October 20, 2010. Available at: https://www.asahq.org/standards-and-guidelines/standards-for-basic-anesthetic-monitoring.

Box 4
Suggested supplies

Airway supplies

  Face masks

  Oral and nasal airways

  Laryngeal mask airways

  Endotracheal tubes: straight and RAE in appropriate sizes

  Stylettes: child and adult

  Laryngoscope blades and handles: various sizes

  Stethoscope

  Suction catheters

Intravenous (IV) supplies

  Cannulas: multiple gauges

  IV tubing sets

  IV buretrols

  Stopcocks

  Sterile dressings

  Tape

  Gauze

  Alcohol wipes

Monitoring

  ECG pads

  Blood pressure cuffs

  Pulse-oximetry probes

  Temperature probes

Personal protective equipment

  Masks

  Hats

  Gloves

  Hand sanitizing gel

---

which includes an assessment of nutritional status and signs of dehydration, especially in hot climates. For patients with cleft lip and/or cleft palate, malnutrition may be present because of difficulties with feeding. Signs of clubbing or cyanosis should be noted and may warrant further evaluation[5] for a possible underlying medical diagnosis. Patient environment may affect patients as well, such as smoke exposure from cooking fires or burning trash. Appropriate laboratory work and radiographs should also be reviewed. It is during this screening process that underlying medical conditions may be diagnosed, including heart disease (unrepaired congenital heart defects,

Box 5
Suggested medications to have available
Volatile anesthetic (sevoflurane, halothane)
IV anesthetics (propofol, dexmedetomidine)
Muscle relaxants (succinylcholine, rocuronium)
Epinephrine
Atropine
Dantrolene
Diphenhydramine
Antibiotics
Narcotics
Local anesthetics
Decadron
Ondansetron
Acetaminophen
Ketorolac
Albuterol
This list is provided for reference and is not intended to be the sole guidance for medications needed.

Box 6	
American Society of Anesthesiologists physical status classification	
ASA I	Normal Healthy Patient
ASA II	Patient with mild systemic disease
ASA III	Patient with severe systemic disease
ASA IV	Patient with severe systemic disease that is a constant threat to life
ASA V	Moribund patient not expected to survive without operation
ASA VI	A declared brain-dead patient for organ donation procedure

From ASA physical status classification system of the American Society of Anesthesiologists. A copy of the full text can be obtained from ASA, 1061 American Lane Schaumburg, IL 60173-4973 or online at https://www.asahq.org/standards-and-guidelines/asa-physical-status-classification-system

rheumatic heart disease, and so forth), pneumonia, or a common upper respiratory infection.

The anesthesia providers should consider undiagnosed syndromes in pediatric patients that could pose an increased anesthetic risk. For example, patients with Pierre Robin sequence could present difficulties with intubation and might not be appropriate patients without additional airway equipment. Given that surgical procedures are most likely elective, the determination of an increased anesthetic risk means the procedure should be deferred. For such procedures that might benefit from additional equipment, the local hospital could maintain contact with the patient so that future surgical teams could arrange to transport the needed equipment for the potential difficult airway. In patients with an unrepaired congenital heart defect, an explanation of surgical and anesthesia risk should be done with the use of an interpreter if needed and the surgery deferred. The patient should be referred to a center capable of cardiac surgery for further care.

There are several additional factors to consider during patient selection. Having appropriate medical translators is important so that an accurate history as well as a well-informed consent can be completed. Be aware that families may conceal medical issues to avoid cancellation of surgery,[1] thereby complicating the process of patient selection. Also, there should be consideration to do procedures with patients of ASA status I and II only (**Box 6**).

Musgrave Rule of 10s

The often-used guidelines for cleft lip and palate repair include weight more than 4.5 kg (10 pounds), hemoglobin level more than 10 g/dL, white blood count less than 10,000/μL,[6] and age more than 10 weeks. Chow and colleagues[6] evaluated the utility of this rule of 10s in relation to adverse outcomes and found there was no justification for the adoption of these guidelines. The study mentioned that procedures were done in the United States with improvement in anesthesia care and postoperative care for pediatric patients. In a low-resource setting without similar standards, minimal adverse outcomes may not be achievable. In the absence of any guidance, the Musgrave rule of 10s remains a reasonable tool for patient selection but probably should not be strictly enforced if other criteria make the patient a suitable surgical candidate. The surgical team should consider adverse outcomes on previous surgical mission trips for possible adjustment to selection criteria moving forward.

Preoperative Fasting

The ASA fasting guidelines are shown in **Table 1** for reference when scheduling procedures.[10] Ensure that patient families have a good understanding of nil-by-mouth policy and the risks of not adhering to the fasting guidelines.

Table 1
American Society of Anesthesiologists fasting guidelines

Type of Food	Time (h)	Example
Clear liquids	2	Water, apple juice
Breast milk	4	—
Nonhuman milk	6	Cow's milk
Formula	6	Infant formula
Light meal	6	Toast, nonfatty
Solid food	8	Fatty meal

Data from Practice guidelines for preoperative fasting and the use of pharmacologic agents to reduce the risk of pulmonary aspiration: application to healthy patients undergoing elective procedures: an updated report by the American Society of Anesthesiologists Task Force on Preoperative Fasting and the Use of Pharmacologic Agents to Reduce the Risk of Pulmonary Aspiration. Anesthesiology. 2017;126(3):376–93.

INTRAOPERATIVE MANAGEMENT

Premedication is rarely available for preoperative anxiolysis, but it can be beneficial in some cases. If a parent or guardian is available to hold the child for induction, this can help ease anxiety in the absence of premedication. The commonly used medications and dosages for oral (PO), IV, and intramuscular (IM) dosing are shown in **Table 2**. Notably, ketamine has a side effect of secretions that can be prevented with addition of atropine in the IM dose.

INDUCTION AND AIRWAY MANAGEMENT

Induction of anesthesia and airway management is of critical importance to patient safety. For surgeries in pediatric patients, most inductions are done with inhalational anesthetics. Sevoflurane is the most commonly used inhalational anesthetic in most high-income countries, but halothane may be the commonly used agent in an

Table 2
Commonly used medications and dosages for oral, intravenous, and intramuscular dosing

Medication	Dose (mg/kg)
Midazolam	PO 0.5–0.7 (maximum 20 mg) IV 0.1 IM 0.1–0.15
Ketamine	PO 5–7 IM 2–3

LMIC. Anesthesiologists unfamiliar with the use of halothane should review its anesthetic properties before use. In older patients with preoperative IV access, an IV induction is preferable to an inhalation induction. Monitors during induction should include noninvasive blood pressure cuff, pulse oximeter, and either 3-lead or 5-lead electrocardiography.[11]

Appropriately sized airway equipment should be readily available during induction (**Fig. 2**). Patients with a cleft lip and/or palate may have a difficult airway and it is advisable to have a second anesthesia provider available during induction and intubation for assistance. If a difficult intubation is anticipated, the emergency airway equipment should be available and the provider should avoid any long-acting neuromuscular blocker. In addition, avoiding routine use of succinylcholine for intubation minimizes any medication side effects.[1] For cleft lip and palate surgeries, oral RAE endotracheal tubes are preferable for optimizing the surgical view and facilitating the use of the Dingman retractor (**Fig. 3**). In addition, a cuffed endotracheal tube provides some protection from aspiration of blood into the lungs during the surgery.

MAINTENANCE OF ANESTHESIA

Volatile anesthetics are used for maintenance of general anesthesia during most procedures. For most procedures, spontaneous ventilation without the use of neuromuscular blocking agents has several advantages. One advantage is that the patient can maintain adequate oxygenation and ventilation if the anesthesia machine stops

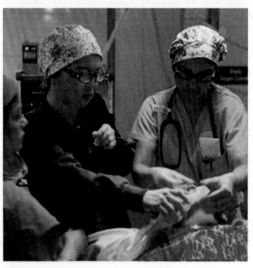

Fig. 2. Anesthesia team securing the airway.

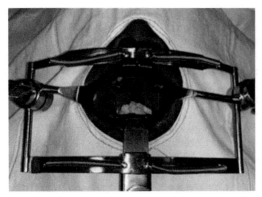

Fig. 3. Dingman retractor in place for cleft palate repair. Note that it is recommended to release the Dingman hourly during surgery to avoid any postoperative glossal edema.

functioning with a power outage. In addition, anesthesia machines capable of mechanical ventilation are infrequently available in low-resource settings.[1] In instances when paralysis is needed, the anesthesia provider can manually provide ventilation if desired when a ventilator is not attached to the anesthesia machine. A twitch monitor aids in determining residual paralysis and the timing for reversal agents.

Pain Management

Pain control consists of multimodal anesthesia, including opioids, adjuncts, and peripheral nerve blocks. If planning to use opioids intraoperatively, it is important to verify what is available within the country because some opioids may not be readily available depending on the location. The anesthesia team should work with the local staff and pharmacy to acquire appropriate narcotics. In addition, they should maintain the standard for disposal and verification of administration. In some cases, the empty narcotic vials must be returned to the pharmacy, so avoid disposal in the sharps container. It is important to remember that controlled medications should not be transported into a country without proper authorization.[1] Adjuncts such as acetaminophen (paracetamol), ketorolac, and ibuprofen are usually readily available compared with opioids. Acetaminophen can be given rectally for infants and children (30 mg/kg per rectum) at the start of the procedure.

Infraorbital Block

For patients undergoing cleft lip repair, a bilateral infraorbital block with bupivacaine 0.25% and epinephrine provides excellent analgesia. This block is performed either transcutaneously or transorally. In some cases, such as cooperative older patients who are not candidates for general anesthesia, local anesthesia can provide adequate operative analgesia for the procedure. If used to supplement general anesthesia, it may be performed either at the start or at the end of the procedure to reduce the need for postoperative opioids.[1]

Throat Packs

Throat packs are placed to reduce the amount of blood and irrigation fluid seeping around the endotracheal tube during the procedure. The use of a cuffed endotracheal tube does not eliminate the need for a correctly placed throat pack. During placement, the endotracheal tube may advance to the right mainstem bronchus and cause a change in oxygenation and ventilation. It is important for the anesthesia provider to ensure the entire throat pack is removed at the end of the procedure before extubation. An inadvertently left throat pack may lead to respiratory compromise in the recovery room if not recognized.

Airway Edema

For cleft lip and palate procedures, dexamethasone is usually administered for airway edema at a dose of 0.5 mg/kg IV (maximum 10 mg). Surgical location, patient positioning, the use of Dingman retractors, and endotracheal tube use all contribute to increased airway edema risk.

Antibiotic Prophylaxis

The use of an antibiotic for surgical prophylaxis is usually accomplished with a third-generation cephalosporin. If there is a suspected allergy, an alternative medication such as clindamycin should be available. The timing and dosage depend on the medication used. The anesthesia team should work with the local staff and pharmacy to determine the medication used for this purpose.

Bleeding

Bleeding intraoperatively is a concern, especially in bilateral cleft lip repair or cleft palate repair. For those cases, careful selection of the patient and preoperative laboratory assessment should have recognized anemia or history of coagulation problems that may create the need for blood transfusion. The availability of blood for transfusion and specific criteria for transfusion should be clear. For other OMFS procedures with a significant risk of blood loss, a type and cross should be in place before starting the procedure.

EXTUBATION

Extubation should occur when the patient has regained protective airway reflexes and shows a return of adequate strength. The anesthesia provider should ensure that the throat pack was removed and airway secretions are minimal. After extubation, lateral positioning for transport to recovery facilitates the draining of any secretions or blood and minimizes pooling in the airway. In addition, lateral positioning can keep the tongue from falling posteriorly and obstructing the airway. For patients with a tongue stitch after cleft palate repair, the tongue can be moved anteriorly to minimize airway obstruction after extubation.[5]

POSTOPERATIVE CARE

There should be adequate nursing personnel in recovery to manage potential airway complications. Local nurses may not be familiar with managing complications, especially in pediatric patients. An anesthesia provider should also be available for any acute airway emergencies. The recovery area should have 1 monitor, or at the least a pulse oximeter, for every 2 patients. Similarly, at least 1 oxygen tank with flow regulator and a facemask should be available for every 2 patients. Suction equipment is also needed in recovery. Emergency airway equipment, including an Ambu bag and resuscitative medications, should be immediately available.

Patients should be maintained in the lateral position in the early postoperative period. Restraints for infants and children should be used to prevent removal of IV access and disruption of the surgical sutures. Careful suctioning of excess secretions and monitoring for airway obstruction or hypoxia should continue until discharge criteria have been reached. Patients undergoing cleft palate repair are particularly vulnerable to airway obstruction caused by airway edema from surgical positioning and the reduced oral cavity with a newly formed palate.[5] The recovery room nursing staff should be familiar with using a tongue stitch to relieve this upper airway obstruction.

Bleeding is a concern in the early postoperative period. Any concerns for excess bleeding in recovery should be brought to the attention of the surgical and anesthesia team. If necessary, plans for surgical control of bleeding should be made so that any available operating table is used during the emergency. If possible, new procedures should not be started so that all available personnel may be available to assist if needed.

Postoperative pain control depends on the procedure and availability of medications. In the case

Table 3
Commonly used medications and dosages for pain relief in the postoperative period

Medication	Dose (mg/kg)
Acetaminophen	PO 15
	PR 30
	IV 10–15
Ketorolac	IV 0.5 (maximum 30 mg)
Ibuprofen	PO 10

Abbreviation: PR, per rectum.

of cleft lip repair, an infraorbital block either before or after the procedure (preferably before extubation) provides excellent pain relief in the early postoperative period.[5] Adjuncts such as acetaminophen (paracetamol), ketorolac, and ibuprofen are usually readily available compared with opioids (**Table 3**). If given intraoperatively, the timing for subsequent doses should be discussed with recovery nurses and local ward staff so as to avoid excess administration. In some countries, pethidine (Demerol), morphine, and fentanyl are all available for postoperative pain control.

Patient families are likely to need education about postoperative recovery and continued patient care after discharge. If postoperative pain medications have child-safe caps, these may be uncommon locally and may need to be explained to parents.

FOLLOW-UP CARE

There should be a well-defined process for managing postoperative issues after hours and after completion of the surgical trip. This process should involve resources of the host country.[1] Any postoperative complications should be addressed promptly. The team should plan a staff wrap-up either at the end of the day or before the start of procedures daily to ensure communication of any updates.

The team should put a quality-assurance process in place to review any events and what could have been done to improve the safety and care of patients.[1]

SUMMARY

Oral and maxillofacial procedures performed in a low-resource environment can be done safely if several factors are considered. The planning and organization should ensure that the appropriate setting, facilities, supplies, and equipment are available, and that the appropriate members of the team are available to provide the perioperative care needed. This team includes anesthesia personnel, circulating nurses, surgical technicians, recovery room nursing, and additional team members such as language interpreters. The anesthesia and surgical teams should determine the types of procedures and criteria for selection of patients before the start of the trip.

The repair of cleft lip and cleft palate remains the most commonly done procedures for orofacial deformities during surgical missions by OMFS providers. Although these repairs can be done at any age, most commonly they are performed on infants and children. The anesthesia providers and recovery room nurses should be comfortable providing care to patients in this age group.

The perioperative management includes appropriate patient selection and determination of anesthesia risk. Intraoperative care is determined by the anesthesia equipment, medications, and supplies available. The surgical team should monitor for any adverse events and make appropriate adjustments to ensure the safety of the patients and a successful surgical trip.

DISCLOSURE

The authors have nothing to disclose.

REFERENCES

1. Fisher QA, Politis GDD, Tobias JD, et al. Pediatric anesthesia for voluntary services abroad. Anesth Analg 2002;95(2):336–50.

2. Khambatta HJ, Westheimer DN, Power RW, et al. Safe, low-technology anesthesia system for medical missions to remote locations. Anesthesiology 2006; 104(6):1354–6.

3. Fisher QA, Nichols D, Stewart FC, et al. Assessing pediatric anesthesia practices for volunteer medical services abroad. Anesthesiology 2001;95(6): 1315–22.

4. Gupta K, Gupta P, Bansal P, et al. Anesthetic management for Smile Train a blessing for population of low socioeconomic status: A prospective study. Anesth Essays Res 2010;4(2):81–4.

5. Gervitz C. Anesthesia considerations for facial deformity repair in lesser developed countries. In: Roth R, Frost EAM, Gevirtz C, et al, editors. The role of anesthesiology in global health: a comprehensive guide. Cham (Switzerland): Springer; 2015. p. 243–55.

6. Chow I, Purnell CA, Hanwright PJ, et al. Evaluating the rule of 10s in cleft lip repair: do data support dogma? Plast Reconstr Surg 2016;138(3):670–9.

7. Jindal P, Khurana G, Gupta D, et al. A retrospective analysis of anesthetic experience in 2917 patients posted for cleft lip and palate repair. Anesth Essays Res 2013;7(3):350–4.

8. Fitzgerald BM, Nagy CJ, Goosman EF, et al. Humanitarian surgical missions: guidelines for successful anesthesia support. J Spec Oper Med 2017;17(4): 56–62.

9. American Society of Anesthesiologists. Standards for basic anesthetic monitoring 2010.

10. Practice guidelines for preoperative fasting and the use of pharmacologic agents to reduce the risk of pulmonary aspiration: application to healthy patients undergoing elective procedures: an updated report by the American Society of Anesthesiologists Task Force on Preoperative Fasting and the Use of Pharmacologic Agents to Reduce the Risk of Pulmonary Aspiration. Anesthesiology 2017;126(3):376–93.

11. Butler M, Drum E, Evans FM, et al. Guidelines and checklists for short-term missions in global pediatric surgery: recommendations from the American Academy of Pediatrics Delivery of Surgical Care Global Health Subcommittee, American Pediatric Surgical Association Global Pediatric Surgery Committee, Society for Pediatric Anesthesia Committee on International Education and Service, and American Pediatric Surgical Nurses Association, Inc. Global Health Special Interest Group. Paediatr Anaesth 2018;28(5):392–410.

Global Nursing in Low-Resource and Middle-Resource Countries
Challenges and Opportunities in Perioperative Practice

Kate Pettorini, MSN, RN, CNOR[a], Mary M. Gullatte, PhD, RN, ANP-BC, AOCN[b],*

KEYWORDS

- Global health nursing • Perioperative nursing • Global surgery • Cleft lip/palate repair

KEY POINTS

- It is important to adhere to ethical principles and guidelines for nursing practice in the global health setting.
- Global health inequities continue to exist, especially in low-resource and middle-resource countries.
- Capacity building in low-resource countries is critical to building a sustainable model of care.
- Global partnerships are crucial in helping to support the World Health Organization, United Nations, and International Council of Nurses goals to improve global health.

INTRODUCTION

The World Health Organization (WHO) and the United Nations (UN) identified sustainable development goals for 2030 for healthy lives and well-being for all by developing a plan to improve global health and to reduce mortality worldwide in noncommunicable disease through medical and surgical intervention.[1] In large part, the impact made in improving global health has been through teams of doctors, nurses, and allied health professionals who often volunteer their time, service, and expertise in the cause of improving the health of humanity.

Traveling to international destinations in low-resource and middle-resource countries is an altruistic way for nurses to serve and to make a difference. It is equally important to give thoughtful consideration to the mission and to plan for sustainability when leaving the country (**Fig. 1**). Gone are the days of going in with the intent of rescuing a situation without leaving behind a sustainable program that can be maintained by the local providers. Capacity building is leaving behind a way to sustain the care by those who live there every day. In addition, it is important to have a working knowledge and understating of the culture and its people. What are their needs versus what others think they need? To this end, global nursing initiatives collaborate with interdisciplinary partners to contribute to the affordable and accessible needed surgical care.

A focus group of expert global nurses conducted a Delphi method to develop the ethical principles and guidelines of global nursing using the International Council of Nurses (ICN) code of ethics as the framework for development of the principles. The outcome of their work was published in *Nursing Outlook* 2018. The nurse experts identified 10 ethical principles of global nursing practice. They also identified 5 domains related

[a] Peri-operative Nursing, 1364 Clifton Road NE, Atlanta, GA 30322, USA; [b] Emory Healthcare Inc, Peachtree Center, 253 Peachtree Street, Northeast, 5th floor, Room 531, Atlanta, GA 30303, USA
* Corresponding author.
E-mail address: mfgulla@emory.edu

Oral Maxillofacial Surg Clin N Am 32 (2020) 437–445
https://doi.org/10.1016/j.coms.2020.04.009
1042-3699/20/© 2020 Elsevier Inc. All rights reserved.

Must do	Should do	Can do
Acute, high-value procedures that need consistency through local structures; and less complex, urgent procedures that can be delivered through these same structures.	High-priority, high-volume procedures for planned surgery at the first-level hospital.	Important procedures potentially needing specialist support. Ideally, higher-risk procedures should be done at tertiary centres, or done at first-level hospitals with the assistance of visiting super-specialist teams.
Acute, high-value procedures include • Laparotomy • Caesarean delivery • Treatment of open fracture	Lower-risk procedures include • Hernia repair • Contracture release • Superficial soft tissue tumor resection • Gastroscopy	Examples include • Thoracic surgery • Transurethral resection of prostate
Lesser complex, urgent procedures include • Wound debridement • Dilation and currettage • Closed fracture reduction	Medium-risk procedures include • Cholecystectomy • Intracranial hematoma evacuation • Thyroidectomy • Mastectomy	• Ureterorenoscopy • Vesicovaginal fistula • Basic skin flaps • Rectal prolapse repair • Cataract • Cleft lip and palate repair

Fig. 1. Common surgical procedures stratified in a must-do, should-do, and can-do framework for first-level care. (*From* Meara J, Leather A, Hagander L, et al. Global surgery 2030: evidence and solutions for achieving health, welfare, and economic development. Lancet 2015;386:586; with permission.)

to ethical guidelines for global health nursing practice. The domains were (1) professional practice, (2) preparation for global health nursing practice, (3) donations for global health nursing practice, (4) global health nursing practice, and (5) evidence-based global health nursing practice.[2] **Boxes 1** and **2** outline these principles and guidelines.

Nurses are at the forefront in volunteering to provide humanitarian health support in local, national, and international disasters. Responding to the call to provide expert medical and surgical education and care in low-resource and middle-resource countries aligns with who nurses are as caring and compassionate professionals.

Most of the current evidence for global nursing work is documented from schools and colleges of nursing with prelicensure students.[3,4] These nursing students often have an elective where they can participate in clinical trips to low-resource and middle-resource countries.

There are marked disparities in supply and demand for specialty-trained health care providers in low-income and middle-income countries (LMIC). Comparing workforce statistics between the United States and developing countries, there are reportedly 253 physicians and 900+ nurses per 100,000 versus 76 physicians and 85 nurses per 100,000 in developing countries.[3] Organizations such as Global Health Service Partnership (GHSP), a public-private partnership between the

US Peace Corps, the US President's Emergency Plan for AIDS Relief (PEPFAR) working to build capacity through professional health education, and Seed Global Health, seek to bring attention to the dire global shortage of health care providers in LMIC. Nursing Now is a collaborative 3-year campaign, with the WHO and the ICN, designed to improve the worldwide status of nurses designed to improve global health. The WHO reports that the shortage of nurses, doctors, and midwives is critical and that, by 2035, the shortage of these professionals will approach 12.9 million in LMIC. The global work to help build medical capacity is crucial (Tefera G, unpublished data, 2017).[5]

GLOBAL SURGERY INITIATIVE: A MISSION TO RESTORE SMILES

More than 70% of the world's population lacks access to restorative, safe, and affordable surgical care, particularly in LMIC.[6] It is reported that "the burden of untreated surgical disease is largely borne by the world's poor."[7] In rural areas in LMIC, the low provider/population ratio of surgeons able to perform lifesaving surgical procedures includes perioperative nurses who provide supportive perioperative care and education.[3] In addition to a shortage of skilled providers, other complex barriers exist preventing patients from accessing safe surgical care when needed, or

---

Box 1
Ethical principles of global health nursing practice

1. The global health nurse promotes an environment in which the human rights, dignity, values, customs, and spiritual beliefs of the individual, family, and community are respected. (0.90)

2. The global health nurse advocates for equality and social justice in resource allocation, access to health care and other social and economic services (ICN, 2012). (0.76)

3. The global health nurse shows professional values such as respectfulness, responsiveness, compassion, trustworthiness, and integrity (ICN, 2012). (0.92)

4. The global health nurse values diversity of opinion, beliefs, culture, and perspectives. (0.88)

5. The global health nurse consistently maintains standards of personal conduct that reflect well on the profession and enhance its image and public confidence (ICN, 2012). (0.77)

6. The global health nurse strives to foster and maintain a practice culture promoting ethical behavior and open dialogue (ICN, 2012). (0.77)

7. The global health nurse must show responsibility and accountability for nursing practice and for maintaining competence by continual learning (ICN, 2012). (0.79)

8. The global health nurse strives to promote safe working conditions for nurses globally. (0.74[a])

9. The global health nurse sustains a collaborative and respectful relationship with coworkers in nursing and other fields (ICN, 2012). (0.81)

10. The global health nurse works in partnership with host country nurses, groups, and governmental and nongovernmental organizations. (0.79)

Numbers in parentheses indicate the item content validity index (I-CVI) value.[a] Indicates that the ethical principle was judged important by the panel of global health nurse experts.
From McDermott-Levy R, Leffers J, Mayaka J. Ethical principles and guidelines of global health nursing practice. Nurs Outlook 2018;66:477; with permission.

---

facing financial ruin to attain it.[6] Barriers to surgical care also include health literacy, lack of access to surgical centers, anesthesiologist, and financial toxicity).[8]

Cleft lip with or without cleft palate is a common birth defect affecting the lip, nose, and oral cavity that requires specialized surgical skill to repair[9] (**Figs. 2–4**). Children born with this condition have difficulty eating, talking, and even breathing until the defect can be repaired. These children often face social stigmas, and endure ridicule and isolation. There can be long-lasting consequences, psychological, emotional, and physical, when a cleft lip and/or palate is left untreated.[10] In LMIC, few surgeons are present who are trained to repair this defect. This need has in small part been met by specialized visiting surgical teams.[6]

CASE STUDY: TRAVELING WITH A TEAM THROUGH A NONPROFIT ORGANIZATION

In preparation for a surgical outreach program to provide care to children with cleft lip and cleft palate birth defects in LMIC, an interdisciplinary team of volunteers is assembled. This case study reflects 1 team's journey. The team includes surgeons, nurses, anesthesia providers, surgical and anesthesia technicians, speech therapists, administrators, and nonclinical volunteers. Before departure to the destination, a briefing, or orientation, is conducted with new and experienced team members. Discussion includes:

- Meet and greet among team members
- Culture of host country residents
- Geography of region
- Required immunizations for the region
- Personal and public safety considerations
- Emergency preparedness
- Overview of workflow, including setup of the operating room (OR), preoperative and postoperative areas, supply storage, case turnover, instrument and supply use, sterilization of instruments, and collaboration with local hospital staff

Supplies are gathered through multiple sources, including donations from local US nonprofits as well as industry partners. Monetary donations provided through the sponsoring nonprofit are used to purchase any additional supplies needed from the host country, such as medications or additional OR supplies.

This mission trip is sponsored by the Rotary Club in Santa Cruz, Bolivia, in partnership with

Box 2
Ethical guidelines for global health nursing practice

Professional practice

1. The global health nurse consistently acts in a professional manner. (0.92)

2. The global health nurse responds according to the scope and standards of nursing practice, including the nursing code of ethics (ICN, American Nurses Association, and host country). (0.79)

3. The global health nurse follows the principles of nonmaleficence (first do no harm) to promote safe and healthy health care environments. (0.89)

4. The global health nurse maintains ethical standards for personal conduct with people in all global health settings. (0.89)

5. The global health nurse is committed to personal and professional growth in maintaining and enhancing competencies in clinical, education, research, and/or administrative practice. (0.75)[a]

6. The global health nurse maintains professional, respectful, and caring relationships/interactions characterized by integrity, honesty, and transparency when dealing with international patients, colleagues, and communities. (0.91)

7. The global health nurse maintains healthy and culturally appropriate behavior with regard to communication, dress, judicious use of alcohol, medication, and other substances, and follows safe sexual practices. (0.81)

8. The global health nurse ensures personal safety and the safety of others while participating in travel associated with nursing practice in international settings. (0.80)

9. The global health nurse respects the economic and resource status of host country populations in communication and use of material resources while in global health settings. (0.69)[a]

10. The global health nurse upholds ethical standards for the nurse and those to whom care is delegated to ensure patient safety and quality of care. (0.87)

11. The global health nurse holds in confidence personal information and uses judgment in sharing this information (ICN, 2012) within the cultural norms of the setting. (0.82)

12. The global health nurse adheres to ethical guidelines for informed consent for patients who agree to nursing assessments and treatments with emphasis on doing no harm. (0.82)

13. The global health nurse ensures that the use of technology such as shared Internet sites, social media, photographic images, and audio and video recordings adheres to informed consent, privacy, dignity, and the rights of people. (0.82)

14. The global health nurse adheres to ethical guidelines for informed consent and protection of human subjects for research that is consistent with the regulations of the home country and institution and national regulations of the host setting. (0.89)

Preparation for global health nursing practice

1. The global health nurse prepares to visit an international setting by learning about the history, politics, culture, health, and economic system in that country. (0.72)[a]

2. The global health nurse is knowledgeable about ethical standards of practice in the host setting. (0.72)[a]

Donations in a global health setting

1. The global health nurse is mindful of sustainability and environmental concerns about donations and provision of supplies to international partners and strives to develop solutions with international partners to meet the needs of the community. (0.75)[a]

Global health nursing practice

1. The global health nurse ensures that appropriate approvals, registration, or licensure is obtained in order to practice nursing across international borders (0.76)[a]

2. The global health nurse strives to practice at the highest standard of nursing care within the limitations of resources, training, and adequate staffing. (0.83)

3. The global health nurse respects the culture of the people in the host setting. (0.88)

4. The global health nurse engages in shared dialogue with nurses from the host setting to deepen understanding of local practice and professional issues. (0.76)[a]

5. The global health nurse is honest and transparent when communicating with international patients and communities. (0.83)

6. The global health nurse collaborates with nurses and health professional in the host setting to identify community priorities/needs and cultural practices that may affect health and health care delivery in the host setting. (0.81)

7. The global health nurse strives to develop sustainable host country partnerships with an emphasis on mutual trust, respect, integrity, transparency, and commitment. (0.81)

8. The global health nurse maintain health and culturally appropriate behavior with regard to communication, dress, and judicious use of alcohol, medication, and other substances and follows safe sexual practices. (0.81)

9. The global health nurse ensures the personal safety and the safety of others while participating in travel associated with nursing practice in international settings. (0.80)

10. The global health nurse upholds ethical standards for the nurse and those to whom care is delegated to ensure patient safety and quality of care. (0.87)

Evidence-based global health nursing practice

1. The global health nurse ensures the protection of vulnerable populations in global nursing research and the application of stringent ethical principles related to the conduct of research. (0.91)

2. The global health nurse meets ethical research standards of the host country regulatory authorities. (0.88)

3. The global health nurse collaborates with host country nurses to advance their knowledge and skill to conduct nursing research and to use research evidence in practice. (0.77)[a]

Numbers in parentheses indicate the I-CVI value.[a] Indicates the guideline was noted as important by the panel of global health nurse experts.
From McDermott-Levy R, Leffers J, Mayaka J. Ethical principles and guidelines of global health nursing practice. Nurs Outlook 2018;66:478; with permission.

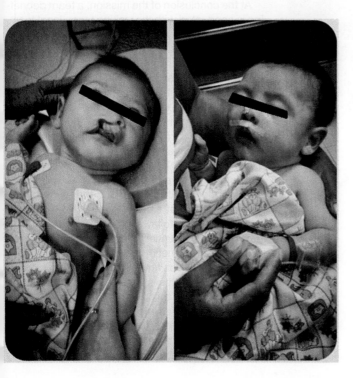

Fig. 2. Cleft lip: infant boy before (*left*) and after (*right*) surgical repair.

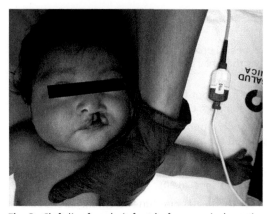

Fig. 3. Cleft lip: female infant before surgical repair.

Healing the Children, Northeast (HTCNE), a nonprofit organization from the United States. Much of the legwork is done by the Rotary Club before arrival of the visiting team. The Rotary Club responsibilities included advertising the mission through multiple media sources, including flyers at local markets, radio, television, and social media, to recruit patients in as many areas of the country as possible. The Rotarians collaborated with local clinics and hospitals to find OR space and resources for the visiting team; communicated the mission with the local ministry of health, customs, and immigration; and provided transportation, information technology resources and translation assistance for the visiting team. Connections are also made with local health providers, including dentists, nurses, surgeons, and students, for an opportunity to participate and learn from the visiting team.

On arrival to the destination, another team briefing is held with the entire visiting team and the local Rotary Club and volunteers. During the meeting, team introductions are made, and there is a discussion of workflow, logistics, and safety, including emergency preparedness for potential events such as malignant hyperthermia crisis, needle stick, and fire, as well as emergency escape routes.

During the week, surgery is provided at no charge to any patient or family. This service includes the cost of transportation and lodging for the family, provided by the sponsoring nonprofit organization in collaboration with the host country Rotary Club. On average, the team performs approximately 50 to 60 surgical procedures over the course of the 1-week mission.

The visiting team works not only to provide patient care but to engage in both didactic and clinical teaching opportunities with the local staff. One or more surgeons will join with the team during the treatment planning and surgical procedures. They are paired with an experienced team surgeon for the procedures. Trainees in all areas are brought in as observers during the perioperative care of the children.

At the conclusion of the mission, a team debriefing is conducted with the visiting team, local team, and Rotary Club members. The entire team reflects on the mission and reviews what went well during the mission and what will make the next mission even better, and there is time for any additional comments from each team member. This process supports the sustainability of the mission, because we learn from each trip and each other and make each mission more successful than the last, strengthening partnerships between the visiting team and host country. Partnering with a local organization and working together to improve each mission has helped lead to the development of a database that can be used to keep track of past patients for follow-up or future care, hoping to close the potential compromise in follow-up care that can sometimes occur after a mission.[11] This team has been fortunate to have the opportunity to return to the same site yearly, starting in 2012, improving training opportunities for local providers as well as providing a reliable team for patients in the area to receive treatment and follow-up care. Children born with a cleft lip or palate birth defect have multiple surgical procedures

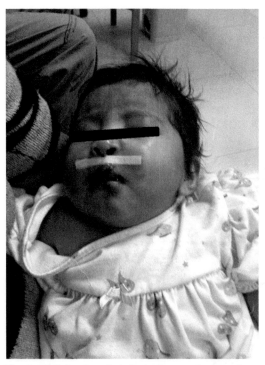

Fig. 4. Cleft lip: female infant after surgical repair.

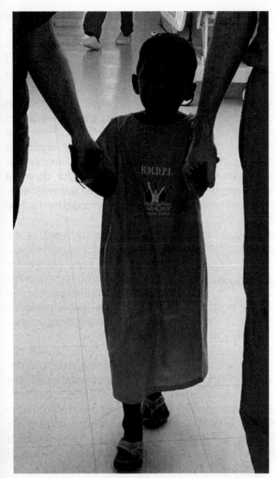

Fig. 5. Child entering surgery suite for cleft palate repair.

throughout their lifetimes (**Fig. 5**). The ability of a patient to be able to rely on affordable, accessible care, can be the difference between receiving treatment versus leaving the defect untreated, suffering all of the associated physical, emotional, and psychological effects.

OPPORTUNITIES

There are many opportunities for nurses to get involved in surgical outreach programs in LMIC, from prelicensure nursing students, who may have an interest or passion to serve the underserved, to experienced nurses who possess the same passion for meeting the health needs other human beings regardless of their social, economic, or health status. There are medical opportunities as well as the surgical global nursing opportunities described in the case study. Making a difference in the lives of children who are often shunned and closed out of their communities

because of the malformation from cleft lip or palate is a journey worth taking. Although there are people who want to make a difference in patient care across the globe, consideration should always be given to ethical principles and guidelines (see **Boxes 1** and **2**). This consideration includes not traveling with preconceived notions of comparisons with how health care is delivered in the United States but accepting where people are and the state of health care and resources in the country being visited.

Visiting a country and providing care is helpful for a short time; however, building capacity among the nursing providers in that country is critical. This process could include mentorship opportunities abroad across all medical and surgical subspecialties,[12,13] including education and training that is linguistically and culturally appropriate to the practicing environment and creating partnerships with hospitals in high-income countries. Nurses can mentor nurses in low-resource and middle-resource countries, keeping up to date with evidence-based practice tailored to their cultural needs and available resources.

Establishing partnerships with nursing associations in the United States and neighboring countries is an opportunity to share education and training materials for further evidence-based development.[4,14] For example, the Association of Perioperative Registered Nurses (AORN) has partnered with the School of Nursing and Midwifery at the University of Rwanda College of Medicine and Health Sciences in supporting a newly developed master of science in nursing program, which offers a specialty track in perioperative nursing. Joining a miniconsortium of nursing associations, AORN has generously donated memberships and educational materials, including the AORN PeriOp 101 program to provide much-needed evidence-based resources to these growing programs.[14] There is an opportunity for visiting perioperative nurses to enhance these collaborations and provide mentorship, training, and education to local staff related to a variety of topics, from evidence-based practice to patient safety guidelines to techniques and procedures.[12,15] Using technology can help sustain these partnerships for mentoring and educating nurses in other cities or countries.[12] Consideration must be made for the learning needs of the local staff, upholding the ethical standards outlined in **Boxes 1** and **2**.

CHALLENGES

At present there are many challenges facing those individuals interested in global nursing. Although it is recommended for specialized teams to support highly specialized surgeries, such as cleft lip and cleft palate repair (See **Fig. 1**), mobilizing a full team takes a coordinated effort. First, the team must have adequate funding to cover flights, housing, supplies, and other costs associated with a surgical outreach program. Team members often use personal vacation time in order to participate in these programs, taking time away from busy practices or jobs at home. Some employers are beginning to support team members by offering other types of paid professional leave, using education or conference hours.

Coordinating schedules can prove to be challenging as well. Surgeons, nurses, anesthesia staff, speech therapists, and other team members must be able to organize a time that also works for the host country, navigating around extreme weather, national and religious holidays, and school schedules to prevent as many barriers to care as possible.

A crucial step to creating a successful surgical outreach program is providing adequate preparation and training for volunteers, from addressing basic logistics such as travel and recommended vaccinations to reviewing the host country's culture, health systems, and other related topics.[11] The nongovernmental organization discussed earlier prepared new and returning volunteers in a discussion format, but this may also be achieved through simulation, case studies, or didactic courses.[11,16] Adequate preparation before an outreach program "equips volunteers with a framework of expectations and tools to process the experiences and challenges."[11(p241)]

MEASURES OF SUCCESS

A picture is worth a thousand smiles. Establishing partnerships within the host country is beneficial in connecting with the ministry of health and providing patient tracking for postprocedure follow-up and new potential cases needing surgery for the next global health visit. The Rotary Club discussed in the case study has been vital in maintaining a partnership in Bolivia. Through this partnership, the program has grown over time, including the addition of a database, maintained by the Rotary Club, which tracks all children who have been screened by our team, allowing easier and more thorough follow-up for future visits. The efforts of the Rotary Club to advertise the program with a variety of far-reaching methods has allowed us to treat children from across the country, including very rural areas.

In addressing the unmet education and surgical training needs of the host country team, it is important to mentor on-site providers in surgical procedures and techniques. This mentoring may include providing lectures, seminars, or hands-on workshops for local providers. Visiting teams can invite local providers to participate in patient care, offering an opportunity for training in surgical techniques and care throughout the visit. Of equal importance is the ability of the visiting health care providers to approach and navigate the host social context with cultural humility.[5] Collaboration with the host team for follow-up and continuing care can ensure optimal patient outcomes. Throughout the year, the Rotary Club provides the visiting team with updates about patients as well as new patients needing care. There is opportunity to further this collaboration through interdisciplinary education for the local surgical, anesthesia, and perioperative nursing teams.

SUMMARY

With a thoughtful, organized, collaborative approach, nurses can participate in fulfilling work in LMIC while helping to improve nursing practice across the world. Working within a framework of ethical principles and guidelines can help create sustainable partnerships that will improve patient care and outcomes globally, in order to meet the 2030 WHO and UN sustainable development goals. For American nurses, working toward improving patient care on a global scale can be extremely rewarding on a personal and professional level.

Nursing participation and contribution to global health can provide a fulfilling sense of pride and a refreshed passion for the nursing profession. However, this contribution is not limited to traveling long distances to care directly for patients. Using technology to provide virtual support for nurses across the world through mentoring, sharing resources, and creating connections through e-mail, Internet, and social media platforms can be very valuable in capacity building.

There has never been a more impactful moment in the authors' lives than watching a mother see her child for the first time after a cleft lip repair. Safe, affordable surgical care should be a right for every global citizen to access when needed.

ACKNOWLEDGMENTS

To the countless named and unnamed nurses and doctors and other members of the surgical teams who unselfishly give of their time and expertise in healing and caring for humanity. To the Rotary Club Sirari in Santa Cruz, Bolivia, and most importantly to Steven M. Roser, DMD, MD, FACS, for his lifelong passion and dedication to improving global surgical care.

DISCLOSURE

The authors have nothing to disclose.

REFERENCES

1. Global action plan. Stronger collaboration, better health. Available at: https://www.who.int/sdg/global-action-plan. Accessed September 1, 2019.

2. McDermott-Levy R, Leffers J, Mayaka. J. Ethical principles and guidelines of global health nursing practice. Nurs Outlook 2018;66:473–81.

3. Pearson A, Jordan Z. Evidence-based healthcare in developing countries. Int J Evid Based Healthc 2010;8:97–100.

4. Upvall M, Trang H, Derstine J, et al. Promoting synergistic partnerships in low resource countries: A case study exemplar. Contemp Nurse 2017;53(5):589–95.

5. Swain J, Matousek A, Scott J, et al. Training surgical residents for a career in academic global surgery: A novel training model. J Surg Educ 2015;72(4):e104–10.

6. Meara J, Leather A, Hagander L, et al. Global surgery 2030: evidence and solutions for achieving health, welfare, and economic development. Lancet 2015;386:569–624.

7. Ng-Kamstra J, Greenberrg S, Abdullah F, et al. Global surgery 2030: A roadmap for high income country actors. BMJ Glob Health 2016;1:e000011.

8. Alkire BC, Raykar NP, Shrime MG, et al. Global access to surgical care: a modelling study. Lancet Glob Health 2015;3(6):e316–23.

9. Mossey PA, Little J, Munger RG, et al. Cleft lip and palate. Lancet 2009;374:1773–85.

10. Sinko K, Cede J, Jagsch R, et al. Facial aesthetics in young adults after cleft lip and palate treatment over five decades. Sci Rep 2017. https://doi.org/10.1038/s41598-017-16249-w. Available at: www.nature.com/scientificreports.

11. Stone GS, Olson KR. The ethics of medical volunteerism. Med Clin North Am 2016;100:237–46.

12. Ibrahim A, Hartjes T, Rivera L, et al. Mentoring researchers in resource-poor countries: The Role of the Clinical Nurse Specialist as Mentor. Clin Nurse Spec 2010;33:7–11.

13. Zaidi M, Haddad L, Lathrop E. Global health opportunities in obstetrics and gynecology training: Examining engagement through an ethical lens. Am J Trop Med Hyg 2015;93(6):1194–200.

14. Mukamana D, Karonkano G, Rosa W. Advancing perioperative nursing in Rwanda through global partnerships and collaboration. AORN J 2016;104(6):583–7.

15. Bickler SW, Spiegel DA. Global surgery- defining a research agenda. Lancet 2008. https://doi.org/10.1016/S140-6736(08)60924-1. Available at: www.thelancet.com.

16. Baumann SL, Sharoff L, Penalo L. Using simulation to enhance global nursing. Nurs Sci Q 2018;31(4):374–8.

Formal Training of the Global Surgeon
Current Educational Paradigms and Critical Elements for Progression

Youmna A. Sherif, MD, Rachel W. Davis, MD*

KEYWORDS

• Global surgery • Training • Medical education • Surgical capacity

KEY POINTS

- Access to safe, timely, and affordable surgical care is an increasingly important global health issue.
- To adequately prepare global surgeons for resource-limited settings, academic institutions have created training programs that provide opportunities to develop foundational clinical knowledge, pursue academic inquiry, build surgical infrastructure and capacity, and become advocates and collaborators.
- Academic institutions can opt to create a short course in global surgery, global surgery rotation, global surgery fellowship, or integrated global surgery residency.
- The creation of a global surgery training program must account for the ethics of global surgery engagement, sources of funding, structures for professional advancement, and partnerships that are trainee appropriate.
- The future of global surgery training must include the establishment of accreditation systems, development of integrated training programs, and institutional investment in global surgery education.

THE EMERGENCE OF A MEDICAL FIELD

Access to safe surgery and anesthesia care is a critical worldwide health disparity and one of the most pressing global health challenges.[1] Unfortunately, surgical capacity building has been historically undervalued because of concerns about prohibitive costs and degree of impact.[2] Research has illustrated that addressing surgical disease burden is a cost-effective global health intervention that has a positive impact in resource-limited settings. Surgical procedures, such as in orthopedics and obstetrics, can surpass the cost-effectiveness of medical interventions, including human immunodeficiency virus treatment. In fact, a significant portion of the global disease burden can be treated with surgical intervention.[3]

The demonstration of cost-effective surgical care in resource-limited settings has emphasized surgical interventions within the global health arena. Major international organizations involved in global health are now prioritizing surgical access and infrastructure. The World Health Organization has emphasized surgical and anesthetic care as part of universal health coverage[4] and the need to develop international surgical and anesthetic guidelines.[5–8] With partners, the World Bank has worked to identify surgeries that are vital to reducing the disease burden in resource-limited settings. As a result, a list of 44 Essential Surgeries that include the fields of general surgery, obstetrics,

Michael E. DeBakey Department of Surgery, Baylor College of Medicine, One Baylor Plaza MS390, Houston, TX 77030, USA
* Corresponding author.
E-mail address: rgwilkin@bcm.edu
Twitter: @youmnasheriff (Y.A.S.); @RachelWDavis (R.W.D.)

Oral Maxillofacial Surg Clin N Am 32 (2020) 447–455
https://doi.org/10.1016/j.coms.2020.04.005
1042-3699/20/© 2020 Elsevier Inc. All rights reserved.

Table 1 The 44 essential surgeries categorized by surgical specialty	
General surgery	Abscess drainage Repair of bowel perforation and peptic ulcer perforation Appendectomy Bowel obstruction Colostomy Gallbladder disease Hernia surgery Fasciotomy Repair of anorectal malformations and Hirschsprung disease
Gynecology	Visual inspection with acetic acid and cryotherapy for precancerous cervical lesions Repair of obstetric fistula
Neurosurgery	Burr holes Hydrocephalus shunt
Obstetrics	Normal delivery Cesarean birth Vacuum extraction/forceps delivery Ectopic pregnancies Manual vacuum aspiration and dealation and curettage Tubal ligation Hysterectomy for uterine rupture and postpartum hemorrhage
Ophthalmology	Cataract extraction and insertion of intraocular lens Eyelid surgery for trachoma
Oral and maxillofacial surgery	Extraction Drainage of dental abscesses Treatment of carries
Orthopedics	Management of nondisplaced fractures Fracture reduction Irrigation and debridement of fractures Placement of external fixators, use of traction Repair of clubfoot Drainage of septic arthritis Debridement of osteomyelitis
Plastic surgery	Escharotomy Repair of cleft lip and cleft palate
Trauma and critical care	Resuscitation Laceration repair Thoracostomy Trauma laparotomy Traumatic amputations
Urology	Vasectomy Hydrocelectomy Relief of urinary obstruction via catheterization or suprapubic cystostomy

Data from Mock CN, Donkor P, Gawande A, et al. Essential surgery: key messages of this volume. In: Debas HT, Donkor P, Gawande A, et al, editors. Disease control priorities, third edition (volume 1): essential surgery. The World Bank; 2015. https://doi.org/10.1596/978-1-4648-0346-8.

ophthalmology, oral and maxillofacial surgery, orthopedics, otolaryngology, neurosurgery, and plastic surgery were compiled in Volume 1 of Disease Control Priorities-3 (**Table 1**).[9] The involvement of international organizations in the standardization of surgical care, development of surgical action plans, and prioritization of safe surgeries has led to a critical and productive examination of the role surgery plays in resource-limited settings.

The conversation about global surgery has continued to evolve within the academic community. It has shifted from short-term engagements to surgical capacity building, training of local providers, and development of surgical education programs.[10] The reconceptualization of surgical care as an international collaboration has resulted in the emergence of global surgery as a medical field. Global surgery is defined as the provision of surgical and anesthetic care to underserved populations in resource-limited settings with the goal of achieving worldwide health equity.[11] In this context, surgical care encompasses the fields of general surgery, obstetrics, ophthalmology, orthopedics, oral and maxillofacial surgery, otolaryngology, neurosurgery, plastic surgery, and urology.

The emphasis on sustainability has necessitated a thoughtful reflection on the global surgeon. The global surgeon has, therefore, been reimagined as an individual who can provide surgical care in a collaborative, community-centered fashion while considering the development of surgical infrastructure, surgical capacity, and the local workforce in resource-limited settings. The global surgeon is therefore not just a skilled surgeon who functions in resource-limited settings. Rather, the global surgeon is an advocate, connector, educator, and ally.

CLINICIAN INTEREST AS A STIMULUS FOR THE CREATION OF GLOBAL SURGERY TRAINING PROGRAMS

One of the greatest driving forces behind the development of global surgery as a field is the tremendous interest expressed on behalf of medical students, surgical trainees, surgical faculty, and private surgeons.[12–14] As this interest continues to grow, academic programs are actively working to break down the multiple institutional barriers to the establishment of global surgery experiences, curricula, and training programs.[15] This movement is fueled partly by a concern about the adequacy of technical, ethical, and scholastic preparedness of surgical trainees for deployment to resource-limited settings.[16] Consequently, academic institutions in high-resource settings have begun developing educational opportunities for trainees.[17–21]

Academic institutions are faced with many challenges as they create global surgery training programs given the relative recency of the field. This is particularly true given the actively evolving definitions of global surgery and the global surgeon. Global surgery training programs are defining the core competencies relevant to the global surgeon, developing longitudinal curricula, establishing meaningful rotations (international and domestic), and structuring the processes for professional advancement in global surgery. Present global surgery training programs are, therefore, simultaneously responsible for the definition of a field and the production of competent global surgeons.

ESSENTIAL GLOBAL SURGICAL EDUCATION AND CORE COMPETENCIES

Global surgery programs must provide their trainees with the opportunities to develop appropriate technical skills to perform common and critical surgeries in austere settings and the foundational knowledge to understand their functions in resource-limited communities. Trainees must be provided with (1) foundational clinical knowledge, (2) skills for the pursuit of academic inquiry, (3) tools for the development of surgical infrastructure and capacity, and (4) education on the nuance of meaningful advocacy and collaborations (**Fig. 1**). In addition, each of these essential tenants of global surgery education must be discussed with a persistent and circumspect consideration of ethics.

Clinical Knowledge

Global surgery trainees should develop a foundational clinical knowledge and exposure to the performance of the 44 essential surgeries and the preoperative, intraoperative, and postoperative management of surgical conditions in resource-limited settings. This training incorporates the exploration of topics not traditionally included in standard surgical training programs. For example, the global surgeon must be trained to manage

postpartum hemorrhage, dental abscesses, open fractures, urologic obstructions, and burn injuries. Additionally, they must acquire an understanding of certain skills critical to the perioperative period that are not typically in the surgeon's purview. An example of this includes the development of ultrasound skills that help guide surgical planning (eg, assessment of gallbladder, thyroid nodules, breast nodules). Similarly, an understanding of performing nerve blockades and delivering spinal anesthesia is exceptionally valuable. This may be accomplished through didactic sessions, journal clubs, and rotations in other surgical subspecialties (eg, obstetrics and gynecology, orthopedics, oral and maxillofacial surgery, urology, and burn surgery).

Academic Inquiry

Within medicine, there is a continuous effort to root interventions and clinical practice in research-based evidence. Therefore, every global surgery trainee should be equipped with the tools to use, understand, and participate in academic inquiry. These tools include a familiarity with seminal articles in global surgery, critical advancements in global surgery, and research methods. It also includes the development of skills, such as grant writing, research design, academic writing, and professional academic advancement.

Surgical Infrastructure and Capacity Building

After establishing essential clinical knowledge and an understanding of academic research, the global surgery trainee must also be educated on becoming a physician-leader. Specifically, she or he must develop a profound understanding of surgical capacity building and infrastructure development because this is one of the most impactful skillsets of the global surgeon. This skillset, in turn, facilitates the appropriate implementation of task sharing and shifting interventions; formation of a surgical team; and development of hospital triage systems, natural disaster plans, and sterilization procedures. This perspective encourages trainees to seek out participation in surgical innovation and equipment design.

Advocacy and Collaboration

Global surgery is deeply rooted in the spirit of advocacy and collaboration. To be active members in such a community, trainees must be familiar with the structure, function, and utility of the international organizations that shape global surgery. Some of these organizations include the World Health Organization; World Bank; International Society of Surgery; World Federation of

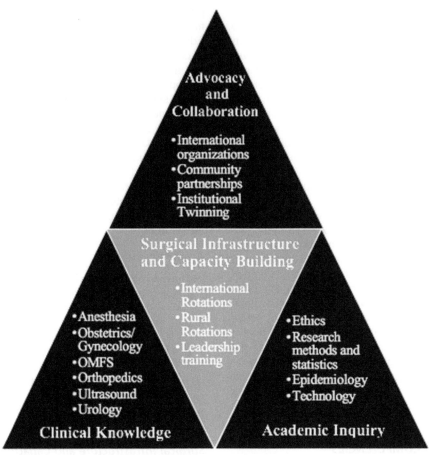

Fig. 1. This diagram illustrates the relationship between the core competencies of global surgery education. The foundation of global surgery education is clinical knowledge and academic inquiry. Surgical infrastructure and capacity building use clinical knowledge and academic inquiry in a real-world context. Advocacy and collaboration, in turn, are skills built on a surgeon's nuanced understanding of critical surgeries in resource-limited regions, enhancement of surgical infrastructure, and advancement of global surgery research.

Societies of Anaesthesiologists; Alliance for Surgery and Anesthesia Presence; Association of Academic Global Surgery; Global Initiative for Children's Surgery; the G4 Alliance; College of Surgeons of East, Central and Southern Africa; West African College of Surgeons; American College of Surgeons; Operation Giving Back; the Royal Colleges in the United Kingdom, Ireland, and Australasia; Resident and Associate Society Global Surgery Workgroup; Incision; and Global Surgery Student Alliance. After understanding this international framework, trainees must develop an understanding of collaboration in global surgery. This includes understanding the importance of community partnerships, reciprocal benefits between partnering institutions, needs assessments, site visits, surgical action plans, and health delivery systems. It is essential to approach global surgery partnerships in a nuanced, culturally competent, and community-centered fashion.

CURRENT MODELS OF GLOBAL SURGERY TRAINING

Academic institutions have proposed and implemented a variety of educational paradigms to provide trainees with the appropriate exposure to the global surgery core competencies. Most of these programs have developed meaningful partnerships with hospitals or academic centers in resource-limited settings. These partnerships are centered on reciprocal contributions, collaborative research projects, and shared goals. The following are the four most common models used at various academic institutions.

Basic Skills Training Course

Academic institutions have created courses that provide medical students, residents, fellows, faculty members, and private practice surgeons with foundational, skills-based training in global surgery.

These courses can last from 1 day to 1 week and include simulations, wet laboratories, and didactics. The skills include the performance of open appendectomies, open cholecystectomies, cesarean sections, incision and drainage of dental abscesses, burr holes, and fracture fixation. The courses may also review certain elements of foundational clinical knowledge, such as ultrasonography and tropical diseases.

Global Surgery Rotation

The Accreditation Council for Graduate Medical Education has allowed credit from international surgical rotations to be applied to residency program completion contingent on the international rotations reflecting the surgical core competencies. As a result, there has been an increase in the number of programs that offer elective global surgery rotations.[22] These electives typically occur in the third or fourth post-graduate year. Most of these rotations occur as reciprocal partnerships between an academic institute in a high-resource region with a partnered academic institution in a resource-limited setting.[21–23] Trainees are able to gain experience in a resource-limited setting and with local faculty. These rotations are intended to offer insight into global surgery and opportunities to help trainees determine their interest in becoming global surgeons.

Global Surgery Fellowship

Academic institutions are beginning to develop global surgery training programs that are pursued after the completion of general surgery residency or during residency research years. In this paradigm, trainees may spend 1 to 2 years at an academic institution concentrating on global surgery research, developing technical skills relevant to global surgery activities, pursuing a master of public health degree, and fostering an understanding of advocacy and establishment of surgical infrastructure. These fellowships allow trainees to spend time learning technical skills and exploring their professional interests in global surgery while receiving appropriate mentorship and guidance from experts in the field. The fellows are afforded the opportunities to spend extended periods of time to truly understand their respective regions of interest.

Integrated Global Surgery Training Program

An integrated global surgery residency track allows trainees to matriculate into standard surgery programs. The trainees in the integrated global surgery track are provided with protected time to rotate through surgical specialties (eg, obstetrics and gynecology, oral and maxillofacial surgery, orthopedics, urology, burn surgery, neurosurgery), pursue global surgery research, and gain experience in global health collaborations and advocacy. Ideally, these trainees are given the opportunity to rotate in Accreditation Council for Graduate Medical Education–approved international rotations during their standard 5-year general surgery training. Additionally, they spend 2 years in pursuit of global surgery projects, training, and research. These experiences are supplemented by a longitudinal curriculum that includes didactics, simulations, and journal clubs.

Other paradigms have been noted in the literature. These include bilateral exchange programs between residencies in high-income countries and residencies in resource-limited settings,[24] fellowships with significant global surgery components (eg, in acute care and global surgery, pediatric surgery and global surgery),[17,25] and integration in military graduate medical education.[26] Ultimately, each training program must determine which model best suits it's institutional values, trainee needs, and departmental vision.

THE PRIMARY CHALLENGES

When creating a global surgery training program it is critical to acknowledge and address the challenges that characterize the field on the individual and institutional level.[12] By recognizing these challenges during the genesis of a global surgery training program, the surgical administration, program directors, chairs, and trainees have the opportunity to strategically plan to minimize the adverse impact of these challenges. Multiple articles have attempted to characterize these challenges and propose thoughtful solutions through strategic planning and adequate preparation.

The Ethical Considerations of Sending Trainees to Resource-Limited Settings

There are multiple ethical quandaries that arise when trainees from high-resource settings travel to resource-limited settings in pursuit of global surgery efforts. These dilemmas are, in part, caused by cross-cultural factors, such as differing ethical frameworks that dictate the bioethics of a region, inability to communicate effectively with patients in their native language, and an incomplete understanding of the cultural context. Similarly, there are ethical concerns about the impact of trainees on resource-limited settings given the less clearly defined structures for supervision, unfamiliar context of care, and conflict with training local providers.[27] Moreover, one must account for the propensity of ethical dilemmas within global surgery even without the added complexity of trainees. These ethical dilemmas include the lack of nongovernmental organization cooperation, pursuit of interventions that are not appropriate to the local community, presence of poorly conceptualized long-term plans, use of technology that is mismatched to local needs, and creation of negatively impactful interventions.[28] Trainees may be left to navigate this ethical terrain without the support traditionally available to them in high-income countries (eg, ethics committees).

Global surgery training programs must attempt to develop rotations that limit ethical concerns, educate trainees on the ethical pitfalls common to global surgery efforts, and provide them with the tools to address ethical dilemmas as they occur in real time. For example, programs can provide trainees with didactic courses on ethics in global surgery with expert lecturers, case scenarios discussed in group settings, and sessions to prepare trainees for their global surgery rotations. Both global surgery training programs and global surgery trainees should develop a systematic approach to addressing ethical dilemmas in global surgery. Such an approach would require the identification of important stakeholders; recognition of perceived medical facts in a particular region; assessment of community goals and values; and understanding of regional legal, ethical, and bioethical standards.[29]

Establishment of Trainee-Appropriate Community Partnerships

One of the most critical components of successful global surgery efforts is the establishment of meaningful community partnerships. Traditionally, this process includes the identification of a community partner, the performance of a needs assessment, creation of a long-term action plan for the training of local providers, consistent outcomes-based monitoring, and establishment of consistent funding sources.[30] In the particular case of global surgery training, the community partnership must allow the trainee to teach and train or be adequately supervised. These sites should also emphasize collaboration with local training programs and the prioritization of training local providers.[30]

Funding

One of the often-cited barriers to the pursuit of global surgery training is generating the finances necessary to support global surgery efforts.[31] For global surgery trainees, it is critical to secure funding for travel, international housing, conference registration fees, vaccination and travel clinic costs,

research, and salaries. Traditionally, a significant proportion of funding for global surgery efforts has been derived from private charitable organizations, government, and aid organizations.[32,33] As global surgery becomes increasingly recognized as an academic field, more funding opportunities are becoming available to trainees (eg, Association for Academic Surgeons Global Surgery Research Fellowship Award, Fogarty funds, Dox Foundation). Global surgery trainees, similar to general surgery residents who pursue 2 years of research, must develop skills in grant writing and fundraising.

Fortunately, academic institutions are beginning to recognize the utility of global surgery training programs and have begun to earmark funds and establish trusts for trainees pursuing global surgery efforts. An academic institution's specific designation of funding to global surgery trainees is reflective of institutional support of these efforts and prioritization of its trainees' adequate preparation for global surgery deployment. This designated funding provides trainees with salary support, which is often not covered by grants. Additionally, designated funding provides trainees with a consistent source of financial support for global surgery efforts. This reduces barriers to pursuit of global surgery training by removing concerns related to the increasing competitiveness of grant applications.

Clear Structures for Professional Advancement in Academic Global Surgery

As academic institutions more completely understand the benefits of global surgery, there is a need to further define a career in academic global surgery. The purpose of this practice is to help the global surgery trainee envision their future careers as academic global surgeons. The academic global surgeon can be described as a physician who has an appointment in an academic center and spends dedicated time, vacation time, or most of their year in a resource-limited setting in a clinical capacity.[34] Responsibilities of the academic global surgeon include the education of trainees, performance of clinical services, engagement in research, and pursuit of advocacy.[35] This may manifest as establishing global surgery rotations for trainees, advising on the performance of needs assessment programs, developing medical education programs, establishing community partnerships for global surgery endeavors, developing cost-effective versions of medical tools, and delivering clinical services to resource-limited settings.[35]

Global surgery efforts are often not considered in academic promotion schemes despite the time and quality of these efforts. Therefore, in addition to defining the academic global surgeon, the parameters for professional advancement in global surgery must also be established. It is presently proposed that global surgery promotion should include certain criteria from the usual promotion track and global surgery-specific criteria.[36] These criteria would emphasize (1) education of trainees in the surgeon's home institution and the partnering institution; (2) research publication in global surgery, weighed equally to other publications; (3) administrative activity in global surgery (eg, development of community partnership, establishment of global surgery tracks); and (4) clinical work at the surgeon's home institution and in the resource-limited setting, valued[36] with potential quantification through global revenue value units. This merging of standard promotion criteria with global surgery activities allows physicians to pursue global surgery without hesitation or fear of career stagnation.

THE FUTURE

The rapid institutionalization of global surgery training programs is, in large part, because of tremendous physician interest, apparent cost-effective interventions, and largely treatable worldwide surgical disease burden. Therefore, this organic, physician-led movement toward incorporating global surgery into clinical practice is derived from the practitioner's desire to be a meaningful contributor, partner, advocate, educator, and champion of safe surgical care and its dissemination. Similarly, the development of global surgery training programs is deeply rooted in trainee passion, faculty mentorship, departmental advocacy, and a receptive institutional culture. The future of global surgery will, in effect, be dependent on and determined by the development of the core competencies, definition of the academic global surgeon, continued investment in global surgery education, and the changing nature of global surgery training given rapidly advancing technology.

Continued Investment in Global Surgery Education

Academic institutions in high-resource settings benefit from a reputation of service, advocacy, research, and education. Global surgery efforts increase the institution's humanitarian profile and allow varied educational experiences for their trainees. International and specialty rotations provide trainees with increased case variety, exposure to complex pathology, understanding of cost-awareness, enhanced cultural competency, and broaden research opportunities.[37] Global

surgery programs increase the marketability of a training program to potential residency candidates. It is, therefore, important for academic institutions to continue to support the efforts of trainees and faculty members.

Development of Integrated Global Surgery Training Programs

Modern trends dictate that the future of global surgery lies in the creation of integrated programs that seamlessly weave surgical specialty rotations, global surgery rotations, global surgery research, and foundational education in global surgery. Trainees will be increasingly able to match directly into a global surgery residency or fellowship program that has a dedicated program director, funding, and established procedures for developing community partnerships. These programs will create technically competent operators that can perform surgeries critical to resource-limited settings across the fields of general surgery, obstetrics, ophthalmology, oral and maxillofacial surgery, orthopedics, otolaryngology, neurosurgery, plastic surgery, and urology. Programs will also provide training in surgical capacity building; creation of surgical infrastructure; establishment of community partners; and performance of global surgery research through didactics, work with international organizations, and participation in community-centered research.

The distinguishing feature of integrated global surgery training is the element of personalized graduate medical education. After completing core competencies, trainees may pursue global surgery efforts specific to their respective interests in terms of region, research, and clinical practice. Ideally, each trainee will be able to create rotations that will best prepare her or him for a future clinical practice as a global surgeon. These opportunities provide trainees with on-the-ground experience establishing community partnerships, needs assessment, creation of surgical infrastructure, and surgical capacity building.

Accreditation of Global Surgery

Accreditation systems ensure that graduate medical education training programs expose trainees to foundational knowledge, comply with current educational standards, and provide critical clinical experiences. Graduating from an accredited program and gaining the appropriate credentialing allows the individual, their patients, their future employers, and their institutions to have a clear understanding of that individual's skillset. This is especially critical in the case of the global surgeon as she or he travels across borders and through various regions to provide safe surgical care to underserved populations. Therefore, there is a need for a system that recognizes competencies and professional certifications in the international setting. It has been proposed that a decentralized global system is optimal because it provides a neutral system for the verification and mutual recognition of medical training and credentialing.[38] Such a system reduces time and paperwork required for licensing when surgeons are traveling across borders, allows for an increased sense of reciprocal and mutual partnerships, and outlines core competencies. A global accreditation system must be housed in a neutral setting, created to monitor case logs and clinical competencies of the individual surgeon, and designed in a user-friendly manner that does not increase the workload of the individual surgeon.[38] The creation of a global accreditation system is a step toward establishing equity among surgeons.

SUMMARY

The creation of academic global surgery training programs is a response to the unmet surgical needs of growing, underserved populations in resource-limited settings. These programs are concerted efforts to produce skilled surgeons who have a shared goal of providing safe surgical care, nuanced understanding of surgical capacity building, and pronounced commitment to building local workforces. The creation of such a surgeon requires the exposure to building surgical infrastructure, refining approaches to academic inquiry in global surgery, and developing a collaborative mentality. This exposure must occur in addition to rigorous training for the necessary technical skills and clinical knowledge critical to surgical work in resource-limited settings. Only then can the global surgeon assist in the delivery of timely, safe, accessible, cost-effective, and locally sourced care. Although tremendous advancements have been made in the development of global surgical training programs, there continue to be challenges to address and areas for improvement. The future of global surgery education is one founded on integrated training programs, meaningful investments in global surgery education, and border-translatable accreditation systems. The future of global surgery education is the creation of the surgeon-advocate, practitioner-capacity builder, and the physician-collaborator.

DISCLOSURE

The authors have nothing to disclose.

REFERENCES

1. Meara JG, Greenberg SLM. The Lancet Commission on Global Surgery. Global Surgery 2030: evidence and solutions for achieving health, welfare and economic development. Surgery 2015;157(5):834–5.
2. Chao TE, Sharma K, Mandigo M, et al. Cost-effectiveness of surgery and its policy implications for global health: a systematic review and analysis. Lancet Glob Health 2014;2(6):e334–45.
3. Shrime MG, Bickler SW, Alkire BC, et al. Global burden of surgical disease: an estimation from the provider perspective. Lancet Glob Health 2015;3(Suppl 2):S8–9.
4. World Health Assembly. Emergency care systems for universal health coverage: ensuring timely care for the acutely ill and injured. Geneva (Switzerland): World Health Organization; 2019.
5. Allegranzi B, Bischoff P, Kubilay Z, et al. Global Guidelines for the Prevention of Surgical Site Infection. Geneva (Switzerland): World Health Organization; 2016. Available at: http://www.ncbi.nlm.nih.gov/books/NBK401132/. Accessed September 17, 2019.
6. Nishiwaki K, Ichikawa T. WHO surgical safety checklist and guideline for safe surgery 2009. Masui 2014;63(3):246–54 [in Japanese].
7. Gelb AW, Morriss WW, Johnson W, et al, International Standards for a Safe Practice of Anesthesia Workgroup. World Health Organization-World Federation of Societies of Anaesthesiologists (WHO-WFSA) international standards for a safe practice of anesthesia. Can J Anaesth 2018;65(6):698–708.
8. Davis RW, Johnson WD. Cross-cutting health: global surgery, obstetrics, anesthesia, and the World Health Organization. Bull Am Coll Surg 2018;103:16–20.
9. Debas HT, Donkor P, Gawande A, et al, editors. Disease control priorities, Third Edition (Volume 1): essential surgery. Washington, DC: The World Bank; 2015. https://doi.org/10.1596/978-1-4648-0346-8.
10. Aliu O, Corlew SD, Heisler ME, et al. Building surgical capacity in low-resource countries: a qualitative analysis of task shifting from surgeon volunteers' perspectives. Ann Plast Surg 2014;72(1):108–12.
11. Dare AJ, Grimes CE, Gillies R, et al. Global surgery: defining an emerging global health field. Lancet 2014;384(9961):2245–7.
12. Cheung M, Healy JM, Hall MR, et al. Assessing interest and barriers for resident and faculty involvement in global surgery. J Surg Educ 2018;75(1):49–57.
13. Scott EM, Fallah PN, Blitzer DN, et al. Next generation of global surgeons: aligning interest with early access to global surgery education. J Surg Res 2019;240:219–26.
14. Johnston PF, Scholer A, Bailey JA, et al. Exploring residents' interest and career aspirations in global surgery. J Surg Res 2018;228:112–7.

15. Fallah PN, Bernstein M. Barriers to participation in global surgery academic collaborations, and possible solutions: a qualitative study. J Neurosurg 2018;1–9. https://doi.org/10.3171/2017.10.JNS17435.

16. Lin Y, Dahm JS, Kushner AL, et al. Are American surgical residents prepared for humanitarian deployment? A comparative analysis of resident and humanitarian case logs. World J Surg 2018;42(1): 32–9.

17. Merchant AI, Walters CB, Valenzuela J, et al. Creating a global acute care surgery fellowship to meet international need. J Surg Educ 2017;74(5): 780–6.

18. Yao CA, Taro TB, Wipfli HL, et al. The Tsao fellowship in global health: a model for international fellowships in a surgery residency. J Craniofac Surg 2016;27(2): 282–5.

19. Donley DK, Graybill CK, Fekadu A, et al. Loma Linda global surgery elective: first 1000 cases. J Surg Educ 2017;74(6):934–8.

20. Esquibel BM, O'Heron CT, Arnold EJ, et al. International surgery electives during general surgery residency: a 9-year experience at an independent academic center. J Surg Educ 2018;75(6):e234–9.

21. Zhang LP, Silverberg D, Divino CM, et al. Building a sustainable global surgical program in an academic department of surgery. Ann Glob Health 2016;82(4): 630–3.

22. Knudson MM, Tarpley MJ, Numann PJ. Global surgery opportunities for U.S. surgical residents: an interim report. J Surg Educ 2015;72(4):e60–5.

23. Hoehn RS, Davis BR, Huber NL, et al. A systematic approach to developing a global surgery elective. J Surg Educ 2015;72(4):e15–20.

24. Baird R, Poenaru D, Ganey M, et al. Partnership in fellowship: comparative analysis of pediatric surgical training and evaluation of a fellow exchange between Canada and Kenya. J Pediatr Surg 2016; 51(10):1704–10.

25. Aarabi S, Smithers C, Fils M-ML, et al. Global Surgery Fellowship: a model for surgical care and education in resource-poor countries. J Pediatr Surg 2015;50(10):1772–5.

26. Jensen S, Tadlock MD, Douglas T, et al. Integration of surgical residency training with US military humanitarian missions. J Surg Educ 2015;72(5): 898–903.

27. Steyn E, Edge J. Ethical considerations in global surgery. Br J Surg 2019;106(2):e17–9.

28. Schein M. Seven sins of humanitarian medicine. World J Surg 2010;34(3):471–2.

29. Wall AE. Ethics in global surgery. World J Surg 2014; 38(7):1574–80.

30. Grimes CE, Maraka J, Kingsnorth AN, et al. Guidelines for surgeons on establishing projects in low-income countries. World J Surg 2013;37(6):1203–7.

31. Chao TE, Riesel JN, Anderson GA, et al. Building a global surgery initiative through evaluation, collaboration, and training: the Massachusetts General Hospital Experience. J Surg Educ 2015;72(4):e21–8.

32. Gutnik LA, Yamey G, Dare AJ, et al. Financial contribution to global surgery: an analysis of 160 international charitable organisations. Lancet 2015; 385(Suppl 2):S52.

33. Gutnik LA, Dielman J, Dare AJ, et al. Funding flows to global surgery: an analysis of contributions from the USA. Lancet 2015;385(Suppl 2):S51.

34. Rickard J, Onwuka E, Joseph S, et al. Value of global surgical activities for US Academic Health Centers: a position paper by the association for academic surgery global affairs committee, Society of University Surgeons Committee on Global Academic Surgery, and American College of Surgeons' Operation Giving Back. J Am Coll Surg 2018;227(4): 455–66.e6.

35. Krishnaswami S, Stephens CQ, Yang GP, et al. An academic career in global surgery: a position paper from the Society of University Surgeons Committee on Academic Global Surgery. Surgery 2018;163(4): 954–60.

36. Wren SM, Balch CM, Doherty GM, et al. Academic advancement in global surgery: appointment, promotion, and tenure. Ann Surg 2020;271(2):279–82.

37. Kang D, Siddiqui S, Weiss H, et al. Are we meeting ACGME core competencies? A systematic review of literature on international surgical rotations. Am J Surg 2018;216(4):782–6.

38. Stawicki SP, Nwomeh BC, Peck GL, et al. Training and accrediting international surgeons. Br J Surg 2019;106(2):e27–33.

Answering the Call
How to Establish a Dentoalveolar Surgery Mission in Low- and Middle-Income Countries

Victoria A. Mañón, DDS[a], Nagi Demian, DDS, MD[a],
Shahid R. Aziz, DMD, MD, FRCS(Ed)[b,c,d,e], Jose M. Marchena, DMD, MD[d,e,f],*

KEYWORDS

- Dentoalveolar • Mission trip • Low- and middle-income countries • Clinical workflow
- Clinical design • Humanitarian aid • Mission ethics

KEY POINTS

- According to the World Health Organization (WHO), approximately 93% of WHO member nations have less than 1 dentist per population of 1000 people, leading to tremendous discrepancies in access to oral health care.
- Identifying a population to serve and providing necessary dentoalveolar services may provide short-term alleviation for those without access to care.
- Designing an international mission requires months of meticulous planning, including communication with the locals, identifying worksites, designing clinic layouts and workflows, team preparation, collection of supplies, fundraising, and advertising.
- Ethical considerations when delivering care in a foreign country must be considered, including patient privacy, informed consent, avoiding exploitation of vulnerable populations, offending local hosts, need for data collection, and sustainability.

INTRODUCTION

According to the World Health Organization (WHO), oral diseases are the most common noncommunicable diseases in the world, affecting 3.58 billion people worldwide.[1] Oral health diseases include dental caries, periodontal disease, oral cancer, dental and maxillofacial trauma, oral manifestations of HIV/HPV, and cleft lip and palates.[2–5] These diseases can affect people throughout their lives, causing "pain, discomfort, disfigurement, and even death."[6] It is estimated that more than half the world's population suffers from dental caries and periodontal disease is estimated to be the 11th most common cause of tooth loss globally.[1] In some regions of the world, such as certain Asian-Pacific countries, oral cancer is in the top 3 most common cancers.[7] In addition to the global prevalence of oral and maxillofacial diseases, there are tremendous disparities in access to dentoalveolar care around the world.[8,9]

[a] Oral and Maxillofacial Surgery, Department of Oral and Maxillofacial Surgery, University of Texas Health Science Center at Houston, School of Dentistry, 7500 Cambridge Street, Suite 6510, Houston, TX 77054, USA; [b] Department of Oral and Maxillofacial Surgery, Rutgers School of Dental Medicine, 110 Bergen Street, Room B854, Newark, NJ 07101-1709, USA; [c] Division of Plastic and Reconstructive Surgery, Department of Surgery, Rutgers – New Jersey Medical School, Newark, NJ, USA; [d] Update Dental College, Dhaka, Bangladesh; [e] Smile Bangladesh; [f] Department of Oral and Maxillofacial Surgery, The University of Texas Health Science Center at Houston, Ben Taub Hospital, Houston, TX, USA
* Corresponding author. UT Oral and Maxillofacial Surgery, Scurlock Tower, Suite 1900, 6560 Fannin Street, Houston, TX 77030.
E-mail address: Jose.M.Marchena@uth.tmc.edu

Oral Maxillofacial Surg Clin N Am 32 (2020) 457–470
https://doi.org/10.1016/j.coms.2020.04.007

Numerous factors contribute to oral health disparities in countries of low and middle socioeconomic status including shortages of medical personnel, limited resources, and limited facilities.[9] In industrialized countries, the average dentist-to-population ratio is approximately 1:2000; in other countries, the ratio is much smaller.[10] Although the average ratio of dentists to population in Africa is 1:150,000, countries such as Ethiopia have a ratio of 1:1,300,000. The ratios of other countries across the globe are equally concerning, with Haiti's ratio at 1:160,000, and rural India at 1:300,000.[11] As a result of inaccessible care, oral health diseases disproportionately affect those of lower socioeconomic status.[8] Many of the oral diseases observed in such populations are preventable and begin to emerge in childhood, and persist throughout the person's life. Even with access to care, health facilities may not be sufficiently equipped to manage many conditions and limit their services to oral prophylaxis and emergency care.[10]

There is a tremendous need for intervention, and each contribution has the potential to make a lasting and meaningful impact. As experts of oral and maxillofacial diseases, oral surgeons are able to help improve access to oral surgical care through humanitarian international missions. Collaborative efforts with general dentists, other specialists, or other surgeons can help provide necessary personnel and supplies to deliver treatment. The objective of this review is to provide the interested surgeon with practical information about how to organize an international mission trip and provide routine oral surgical care in a foreign low- and middle-income population rural setting.

CHOOSING A POPULATION AND ESTABLISHING LOCAL CONTACTS

When choosing a population to be served by a mission, it is important to take several factors into consideration. These factors include evaluation of the team's capacity, the considered population's needs, locals' attitudes toward foreign intervention, interpersonal connections between mission teams and foreign institutions/contacts, and capacity for patient follow-up.[11]

First, a thorough evaluation of the services the team is able to provide is critical. A list of potential routine oral surgical treatments is presented in **Box 1**. Attempting to provide a medical service that a population needs, but for which the team is not prepared to deliver, may result in avoidable treatment complications and long-term harm. The inability to provide services may result from incompetence in a specific surgical skill set, a

---

> **Box 1**
> **A list of oral surgical procedures that may be delivered during a mission trip**
>
> - Routine and surgical dental extractions
> - Alveoloplasty
> - Incision and drainage of abscesses
> - Incisional and excisional biopsies
> - Removal of foreign bodies or bony spicules
> - Assessment and treatment of dentoalveolar trauma
> - Pediatric oral surgery
> - Head and neck cancer screening

---

lack of supplies or equipment, or lack of supporting personnel. During this evaluation, team leaders should identify the needs of the people they plan to serve and compare their needs with the providable services. This will guide the formation of the team and acquisition of equipment. This also prevents accumulation of unneeded equipment/supplies, communicates the need for treatment boundaries to the other team members, and reduces the risk of patient complications.[12]

The evaluation of the populations' needs is very important because providing an unneeded service adds unnecessary costs for the team and does more harm than good to the local people and economy. For instance, if a mission team is able to provide a specific service for a population, but local practitioners are also able to provide that same service, the transient loss of patients may result in financial distress for the local practitioners and economy. If the said service is unavailable or inaccessible, only then should the team consider intervention. In other words, just because a service can be provided does not mean that it should. Although the aim of a mission trip is to help others, it should not be at the expense of the local economy.[13] Providing services that are needed and inaccessible results in a win-win-win situation for the mission team, the patients, and the economy that regains healthier members who can now better contribute.[14]

Local perceptions of foreign help should also be evaluated when selecting a community, because development of a healthy relationship among the mission team and locals is critical for success. Certain populations are not as open to accepting foreign aid as others; these cultural influences should not be ignored because entering communities where the team is not welcome can be dangerous and may incite conflict. Foreign governments may view foreign aid as a form of exploitation or a means to create dependency on the providing country.[15] Safety of the mission team should be a primary consideration, and a location should be chosen where the locals and the teams' values are correlated.[16–18] Although local ideologies and customs may differ from the those of the team, these differences should be respected, promoting collegiality and partnership among the team and the locals.[13]

How, then, does one develop an international relationship with the intention of establishing a mission trip? Foreign connections can be made through existing personal connections, through institutions (religious and academic), or through existing nonaffiliated mission groups. Personal contacts with ties to an existing international network can facilitate the process of meeting partners in foreign countries who may have knowledge of populations with limited access to care or an understanding of the local policies. Standing institutions are often havens for outreach and may provide access to international contacts. Many religious groups, including churches, often provide funding for their members or establish teams. In academia, there has been a tremendous push for the establishment of global surgery as a subspecialty, advocating for research and development of foreign training programs.[19] Nonprofit, nonreligious groups may also provide opportunities, such as International Medical Relief, Mission to Heal, and Doctors Without Borders, to name a few. The American Dental Association provides a trip calendar for interested volunteers.[20]

Finally, once a population has been identified, the team needs to plan for follow-up care after the completion of the mission. If the team maintains consistent operations throughout the year, patients may continue to follow up with the team. If the team is only available annually or seasonally, ensuring that the local population has a way to manage complications is paramount. While building connections with the local population, it is extremely beneficial to identify local practitioners who may be able to assist in the mission. This may include using a local hospital or clinic as a primary site of operation, or recruiting local practitioners to volunteer their services. If it is not possible to establish follow-up care for patients, the team should consider alternative options. The purpose of the mission should be to have good outcomes and leave the patients healthier after the treatment and to avoid complications that may have not otherwise occurred without intervention. Measuring of treatment outcomes should be incorporated into the paradigm of the mission; these data will assist with quality improvement and can be disseminated to help expand the inadequate body of literature.[21,22]

RESERVING A WORKSITE AND DETERMINING AVAILABLE RESOURCES

Once a population has been identified and local contacts are established, the logistical planning of the mission begins. Planning prevents waste and unnecessary expenses.[13] This includes evaluation of the worksite, establishment of clinic workflow, development of a work schedule, recruitment and preparation of team members, and fundraising.[11,23] The importance of clear and constant communication cannot be overemphasized; although changes and unexpected events may occur, maintaining communication with the local contacts, the team, and other coleaders during the planning process will help mitigate unanticipated setbacks.

Evaluation of the Worksite and Determining Needed Supplies

When possible, team leaders should visit the worksites to determine the availability of space (land), equipment, and supplies at the site(s). Land will include the site's infrastructure, including the building, number of dental chairs, and space available for waiting patients and postoperative recovery. Equipment includes radiology and sterilization equipment, surgical instruments, and emergency crash carts.[23,24] A checklist of necessary supplies is presented in **Box 2**. In addition to surgical supplies, other necessary supplies may include tarps, rope, and conventional chairs, to name a few (**Fig. 1**).[23] These items can often be found and purchased in the country. If the mission leader is unable to visit the site before planning or departure, close communication with the local contact is crucial.[11] Items not available at the site will need to be brought by the team.

Availability of space, equipment, and supplies, in addition to the duration of the mission trip, will help determine the services that may be reasonably provided, the number and type of team members needed, and the number of patients that can be treated. This information will guide the creation of itemized supply logs, determine the funds needed to obtain necessary supplies, team recruitment applications, and the design of clinic layout and flow. Setting fundraising goals and providing itemized spreadsheets will also help obtain donations because donors often seek verification that their contribution is appropriately used.[11,21]

Box 2
Comprehensive list of oral and maxillofacial surgical supplies

Disposable Surgical Supplies

- Gauze (4 × 4 and 2 × 2; additional supply to send home with patients)
- Mirrors
- Surgical towels or patient bibs
- Syringes
- Needles
- Penrose drains
- Sutures (dissolvable recommended)
- Cotton tip applicators
- Tongue depressors
- Size 15 blades
- Saline or sterile water (preferably purchased in the country because this is heavy to transport)
- Suction tips
- Disposable cups for expectorants

Medications

- Pain medications[a]
- Antibiotics[b]
- Local anesthetics (with and without epinephrine)
- Peridex mouth rinse

Personal Protective Equipment

- Magnification loupes or protective eyewear
- Gowns
- Surgical masks
- Surgical gloves
- Surgical caps and bouffants
- Scrubs
- Shoe covers
- Sharps containers

Nondisposable Surgical Supplies (Surgical Tray)

- Blade handle[c]
- Periosteal elevator[c]
- Scissors[c]
- Hemostats[c]
- Pickups[c]
- Needle drivers[c]
- Basin[c]
- Syringe[c]
- Curettes[c]
- Minnesota retractor[c]
- Elevators[c]
- Mirror[c]
- Bite block[c]

- Rongeurs[c]
- Handpiece with burs
- Forceps (assortment and personal preference is recommended; 150, 151, 23)
- Root tip picks

Sterilization/Sanitation Equipment

- Sanitation wipes or spray
- Pressure pot cooker with weight
- Sponges or scrubs
- Portable stove top
- Trash bags and waste bins

Emergency Supplies

- Hemostatic agents (gelatin sponges, collagen plugs, tranexamic acid, oxidized cellular polymers, cautery pens)
- Intubation equipment
- Epinephrine
- Sugary beverages (juices, soda)

Other/Miscellaneous

- Portable radiology equipment, including portable x-ray unit, sensors, and laptop
- Blood-pressure cuffs and stethoscopes
- Hand mirrors for patients
- Lubricant for handpieces
- Surge protectors, converters, and adaptors
- Storage containers

This list may be modified to accommodate individual team needs.

[a] Ibuprofen and acetaminophen are medications that can be easily transported by the team. If necessary, local surgeons can provide prescriptions for narcotics.

[b] May need to be purchased in advance because these may not be available for purchase in the country. Alternative options for penicillin-allergic patients are also recommended.

[c] Items to be included in standard tray. Handpieces, burs, and forceps should be used judiciously if fewer of these items are available. Disposable #15 blades with handles may also be preferred.

[d] It is recommended that operations are completed close to a hospital or emergency clinic in case of an adverse event. A standard crash cart should be acquired in the country, if possible.

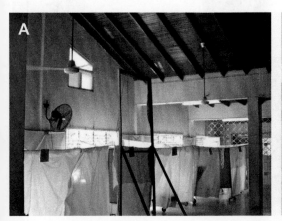
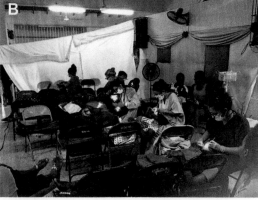

Fig. 1. An improvised clinic in Portmore, Jamaica. (A) Surgical operatories created and separated with sheets and rope to allocate space and ensure patient privacy. (B) With patient consent, foldable office chairs placed side by side were used as dental chairs for examination. (*Courtesy of* [A] Jill Clapp, MSF; [B] Megan Luna, RDH).

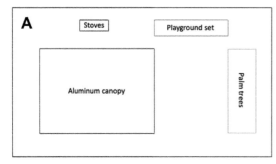
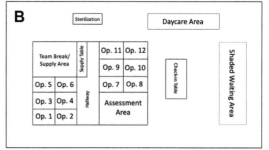

Fig. 2. (*A, B*) Utilization of buildings and equipment in a recreational park in Lauriston, Jamaica. (*Courtesy of* Victoria A. Mañón, DDS, Houston, TX.)

Designing the Clinic Layout

If no clinic staff or layout is available at the worksite, these should be designed in advance. Before starting operations, the team leader should understand the space layout and construct a functional clinic from the available space and resources (**Figs. 2** and **3**). Space, equipment, and supplies should be used in the most optimal fashion to avoid waste and increase efficiency.[21] These plans detail the physical location of each activity and the supplies, including a patient waiting room, check-

in site, assessment/treatment rooms, recovery rooms, and patient education areas. A clearly designated location for emergency supplies should be determined.[25] Depending on the location, spaces may need to be improvised, particularly if the worksite is in a rural location. Creativity and flexibility are required in these situations because patient safety and privacy should still be of utmost concern. These locations should be clearly labeled at the worksite to promote workflow. Team members should be assigned to operate the areas and should be cross-trained to work

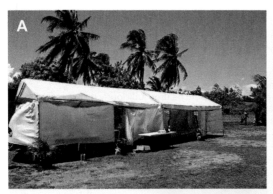
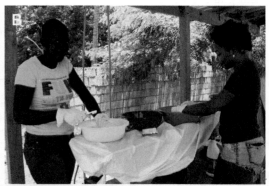
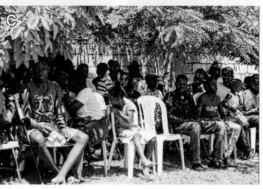

Fig. 3. (*A*) Tarps and sheets were used to separate operatories and assessment areas. (*B*) Outdoor kitchenette space converted to sterilization area. (*C*) Shaded area under trees used as a patient waiting area. (*Courtesy of* [*A*] Megan Luna, RDH; [*B*] Victoria A. Mañón, DDS, Houston, TX; [*C*] Megan Luna, RDH.)

multiple areas. The local population at the mission site may also have personnel available; it is important to communicate in advance so that redundancies in staff are avoided. These plans should be reviewed in advance with the team members. If the local site has an existing layout and plan, these plans should be evaluated and followed according to local policies.

Establishing Clinic Workflow

Once the clinic layout is designed, the clinic's workflow should be established. Clinic workflow describes processes performed by staff and practitioners, and use of equipment that allows efficient treatment of patients. This includes clinical functions and steps that guide the patient's path from check-in, to assessment/treatment, recovery, education, and discharge. Clinic workflow seeks to optimize treatment times and maximize the use of space, supplies, and human resources in the most effective and safe manner. The clinical workflow also includes a tentative schedule of the work days, for example, "Day 1 is an assessment day, Days 2 to 7 are treatment days, and Day 8 is a follow-up day." When creating clinic workflow, team leaders should seek to answer questions such as "Is it more efficient for a patient's medical history and assessment to be completed in a separate assessment clinic or in the treatment chair?" or "If a patient has an adverse event in the chair, such as syncope or an allergic reaction, what precautions have been incorporated into the workflow so that the patient is promptly managed?"[25]

The workflow will define when and where clinic activities will occur and creates designated responsibilities for team members.[26] This prevents missing critical components of patient care, such as obtaining informed consent, and serves as a barrier to prevent complications. An example of a workflow design is shown in **Fig. 4**.

Recruitment and Preparation of Team Members

Once the clinic workflow has been determined, the number of personnel required can be extrapolated. Team personnel include the surgeons and supporting staff, such as front desk attendants, translators, surgical assistants, and other volunteers. Members who are able to assist with translation and patient emergencies should be identified. All personnel should be oriented to the information previously described and will require preparation in advance. Preparation includes discussions on the collection of necessary documentation, clinic and workflow orientation, emergency preparedness training, travel and lodging accommodations, exchange of contact information, and the management of expectations.

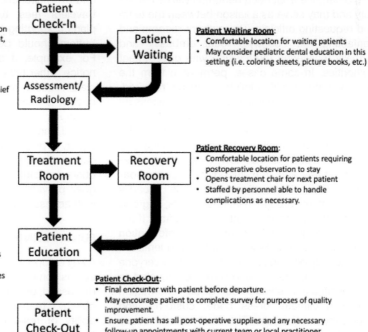

Patient Check-In:
- Establish list of visiting patients
- Complete paperwork including information on patient's name, date of birth, chief complaint, self-reviewed medial/dental history

Assessment:
- Obtain vitals, review medical history and allergies with qualified personnel, discuss chief complaint and HPI.
- Obtain and review indicated radiographs.
- Diagnose patient and treatment plan.
- Review treatment plan with patient/ sign consent form

Treatment Room:
- Review treatment with patient
- Complete indicated treatment.

Patient Education Area:
- Provide post-operative instruction and medications to patient
- Answer all patient questions.
- Promote life style changes and counseling as indicated
- Provide oral hygiene instructions and supplies

Patient Waiting Room:
- Comfortable location for waiting patients
- May consider pediatric dental education in this setting (i.e. coloring sheets, picture books, etc.)

Patient Recovery Room:
- Comfortable location for patients requiring postoperative observation to stay
- Opens treatment chair for next patient
- Staffed by personnel able to handle complications as necessary.

Patient Check-Out:
- Final encounter with patient before departure.
- May encourage patient to complete survey for purposes of quality improvement.
- Ensure patient has all post-operative supplies and any necessary follow-up appointments with current team or local practitioner.

Patient Check-In → Patient Waiting → Assessment/Radiology → Treatment Room → Recovery Room → Patient Education → Patient Check-Out

Fig. 4. Example of a clinical workflow diagram. (*Courtesy of* Victoria A. Mañón, DDS, Houston, TX.)

Recruitment of team members may be accomplished through personal contacts, academic/religious institutions, or social media. Often members will be recruited through "word of mouth," but as the mission is advertised other interested parties may contact the organizing leaders to volunteer. Regardless of physical location, close communication with team members is critical.[11] The committed team members should receive regular updates and be given all necessary information before departure; in turn, team members also need to maintain communication with team leaders during preparation. Recruitment will need to be completed months before departure, and volunteers will need to verify their commitment.

Necessary documentation will need to be collected from the team members and should be submitted to the appropriate local officials. Necessary documentation will vary from country to country and needs to be investigated as soon as the location is determined because some documentation may take months to process. Necessary documentation may include dental/medical licenses, a copy of the diploma, temporary work application forms, a roster of the team including names and stated function on the team, passport information, work visas, and malpractice insurance.[23] If dental students or residents are participating, verification of supervision may also be required.[18] As soon as a team member decides to participate, prompt submission of these documents should be requested. Local contacts can help determine what documentation will be necessary and may serve as a liaison between the team and requesting officials. The authors recommend contacting the country's local embassy and formally registering the mission with government authorities. In some cases, permission from the government's Health Ministry may be required, and the local host should assist with necessary procedures and documentation.

As previously mentioned, the team should be oriented to the details of the mission, including the clinic layout and workflow, their individual responsibilities, and travel/lodging accommodations. This information can be readily communicated through meetings, emails, or group messaging applications such as WhatsApp. If the team is geographically spread out, information may be sent electronically and an orientation meeting may be held on arrival to ensure everyone is prepared. Members who have not traveled to the destination should be given information regarding climate, dress code, customs, and necessary vaccinations. The Centers for Disease Control and Prevention and the US Department of State Bureau of Consular Affairs provide information on travelers' health and travel advisories.[27,28] Contact information of all team members should be exchanged at this time; planning and open communication help ensure the team's safety. Travel and emergency evacuation insurance should be required of all team members. This can be easily obtained through travel or insurance agencies. Malpractice insurance coverage must be considered. For American oral and maxillofacial surgeons, the OMS National Insurance Company will provide coverage for up to 4 weeks of overseas volunteer work. The authors have also used coverage provided by the International Helpers (Guernsey) Trust.

Throughout the planning process, it is important to reassure the team and manage their expectations. Changes in plan will occur and the importance of patience, flexibility, and adaptation need to be emphasized. Team members need to be reminded that they are guests in another country; respect for their culture and policies is mandatory.[11] Additionally, operating conditions may be less than ideal: nonmodifiable factors including weather (particularly when working outdoors), malfunction of equipment and supplies, and/or unexpected events should be handled appropriately. Creativity and innovation are always encouraged.

On arrival into the country, it is important to stay calm and organized. Despite the months of extensive planning and preparation, unanticipated events do occur. Such events may include last-minute withdrawal of personnel, confiscation and/or malfunction of equipment, unexpected travelers' fees, theft, and changes in workday plans. Expecting the unexpected is prudent, and buffers should be incorporated into the plans. For example, if a translator drops out without notice, other team members can translate; if officials request additional fees, a portion of the budget is allocated for emergencies. Global oral surgeons and their teams must be adaptable, ethical, and patient; expression of frustration, anger, or poor character may insult the hosting locals and/or demoralize the team.[11] Despite these obstacles, sight should not be lost of the ultimate goal: providing the underserved local population with access to care.

FUNDRAISING AND ADVERTISING

A key component for mission success includes the acquisition of funds and equipment. As previously discussed, determining which services are providable by a team is partially determined by the availability of resources; this includes the group's finances. To increase the team's financial resources, fundraising and advertising are important aspects of planning the mission trip. These efforts serve a dual purpose: they educate donors and the community about the health care disparities across the world, and encourage them to participate in the efforts through their contributions.

Funding can be obtained from various sources, including self-funding, individual and company donations, and grant agencies, and also through sales; the overall budget is likely composed of a combination of these. As a mission trip is initially formed, the mission leaders may need to invest their own financial resources into the group, which may ensure that the mission is successful in its infancy.[19] Missions may also receive money or supplies from individual donors or from for-profit companies. Individuals aware of the cause may choose to donate money to the group; increasing awareness and specifying the needs of the group increase the likelihood of receiving these donations. Targeted fundraising is also useful: reaching out to ex-patriot communities in the United States can be a source of both long-term funding and long-term advertising. Formal requests can be sent to companies because they often allocate an annual budget for charity. It is imperative that these requests are made as early as possible, because companies often receive many requests and their budgets are limited. An application may also be sent to grant agencies, although they often have strict rules about the projects they are allowed to fund. Various grant agencies are listed in **Box 3**; their Web sites may provide more information on what amounts are available and specific qualifications for funding. Lastly, the group may attempt to raise money through sales. The sale of items may also be used to promote the mission, for example through the sale of items with the mission's logo or mission statement, or through the sale of tickets for awareness events. Once funds are collected, the money can be placed in a nonprofit bank account. Nonprofit account status allows donations to be written off as tax-deductible expenses.[29] Nonprofit status (also termed 501c3 status by the US Internal Revenue Service [IRS]) requires a formal application to the IRS.

Advertising should be used to increase awareness of the mission and educate the community about global health care disparities. Target audiences can be reached through personal contacts, social media, fundraising events, and/or through the supporting institution. Effective advertisement clearly communicates the group's mission and project objectives and describes how community members can contribute.[30] Providing photos, videos, and patient accounts can be used to demonstrate that their contribution will make a difference, and providing receipts, itemized checklists, and statistics shows them how they contributed. Flyers, presentations and lectures, published literature, and table booths can also be effective means of advertisement. For these reasons, documentation of mission activities is imperative not only for the purposes of receiving donations but also for the purposes of education.[18] When advertising, it is important to do so in a manner that protects the dignity of the patients and promotes the mission. Posting unauthorized images on social media should be avoided. It is important to avoid exploiting vulnerable populations in the process of raising the funds.[11]

STORAGE AND TRANSPORTATION OF SUPPLIES

Storage and transportation of collected supplies ensures their availability during the mission trip. Storage sites should be identified before departure and at the destination; periodic inventories should be conducted to ensure availability and to identify theft.[31] Because items should be collected well in advance, requesting a volunteer to store the supplies to avoid additional storage costs is ideal. Equipment should be divided into disposable (items that may be left at the worksite or thrown away) and nondisposable (items that will be returned). Nondisposable items must have arrangements for return, especially if they are loaned. Volunteers may be identified to carry on equipment during flights. If transportation costs are incurred, these individuals may be reimbursed at a cheaper rate than paying an independent transporting company.

Nondisposable equipment, such as surgical instruments, handpieces, and radiology and sterilization equipment, must be in working condition

---

Box 3
Humanitarian aid grant agencies

- The Bill and Melinda Gates Foundation
- The Rockefeller Foundation
- The Fogarty International Center
- The Fulbright Scholars Program
- The Carnegie Corporation
- The Wellcome Trust
- National Cancer Institute Center for Global Health
- AAOMS Foundation
- Dollies Making a Difference

and is critical for the success of the mission. As important as these are, equipment is often expensive and may be difficult to acquire. The purchase of surgical instruments and handpieces are usually not within a team's budget, but as the group accumulates funds the team may acquire equipment owned by the organization. This equipment may be used on subsequent trips for the duration of the equipment's life. Equipment can often be loaned by supporting surgeons, dental equipment companies, or institutions. The worksites may also have equipment, but it is prudent to assume that some of the equipment may malfunction or will be unavailable. There should be enough equipment in circulation that allows for operations to continue while contaminated equipment is in sterilization. This ensures efficiency and allows for treatment of a maximum number of patients. For sites that have repeated visits planned, it is helpful to identify a safe and secure storage facility in the country for equipment and supplies.

The local contact should be able to assist with policy information and customs regarding transport of medications and medical supplies. Unless a team member is a licensed professional in the country, it may not be possible to purchase medications; antibiotics and pain medications should be purchased and transported to ensure their availability. Again, communication with the local contacts is imperative when discussing storage and transportation of supplies to avoid theft and confiscation.

INFECTION CONTROL, STERILIZATION, AND WASTE DISPOSAL

Sterilization and sanitation of equipment are equally as important as the surgical instruments themselves. The ability to adequately sterilize instruments and sanitize work stations ensures that patients are kept safe from infection and the transmission of disease.[32] Without these abilities, it is unethical to continue operations. The obligation of the mission is to leave the foreign community in better health than before arrival; failing to complete sterile and sanitation processes is a direct violation of this code.

Personal protective equipment should be made readily available for all personnel working with patients. Gowns, gloves, eye protection, and masks should be worn, even in work environments that are hot and lack air conditioning.[32] It may be necessary to purchase gloves a size larger than usually worn in warm environments to overcome swelling of the hands or perspiration. The team needs to be reminded of the importance of practicing safely and to stay hydrated. Chemical wipes should be readily available and should be used on chairs and work areas between all patients. Sharps containers should be clearly labeled and be placed in every operatory. All hazardous materials should be properly discarded. Given that waste disposal policies may vary from country to country, the local contact should be able to help with disposal of waste.

Although some clinics or hospitals may provide the staff and equipment to sterilize instruments, more rural facilities may not. Alternatively, a stove, pressure pots, and an aluminum ring weight may be used (**Fig. 5**).[23] The weight is designed to apply the necessary pressure to the pot, recreating the pressure of an autoclave. The ring is designed to fit a 4-quart (3.78-L) stainless-steel pressure pot and increases the pressure within the pot from 16 psi to 24 psi, reducing the sterilization time from 15 to 20 minutes to 10 minutes.[23] The weights may be purchased from the Christian Dental Society at their Web site (see **Fig. 5**). If this option is not available, high-level disinfection techniques may be used (**Table 1**) but are not generally recommended.

ETHICAL CONSIDERATIONS

Throughout the planning process, several ethical considerations must be considered. As previously mentioned, the aim of the mission trip is to provide treatment that is standard of care and that upholds the principles of ethics and code of conduct; these principles include patient autonomy, nonmaleficence, beneficence, justice, and veracity.[37]

Upholding patient autonomy includes the process of informed consent. After patient assessment, patients should be informed of the clinical findings, regardless of whether they can be treated

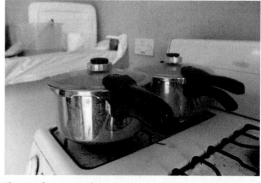

Fig. 5. If an autoclave is not available, a pressure pot with or without a weighted ring may be used to sterilize instruments. The aluminum ring, as seen on the pressure pots, may be purchased at https://www.christiandental.org/sterilization-pressure-pot-ring/.

Table 1
Available sterilization and high-level disinfection techniques

Sterilization Techniques	High-Level Disinfection Techniques
Autoclave: pressurized steam at 15 psi at 121°C for 20–30 min[34,36]	Bleach (5.25% NaOCl) 1:10: dilute with water to reduce Cl concentration; soak for 10 min[33]
Pressure pot cooker without weight: pressurized steam at 16 psi at 121°C for 20–30 min[23,33,34]	Gluteraldehyde: soak for 20–45 min[33]
Pressure pot cooker with aluminum weight: pressurized steam at 24 psi at 121°C for 10 min[23,33,34]	Orthophthaldehyde: soak for 12 min[33] Hydrogen peroxide (7.5% H_2O_2): soak for 30 min at 20°C[33]
Gluteraldehyde: soak for 6–10 h[34,35]	Birex: phenol-based, FDA-approved surface disinfectant[33]
Hydrogen peroxide (7.5% H_2O_2): soak for 6 h at 20°C[33,34]	
Peracetic acid and hydrogen peroxide: powder mixed with water; soak for 10 min[34,35]	

Glutaraldehyde, orthophthaldehyde, and hydrogen peroxide may cause skin, eye, or respiratory irritation; they should not be disposed in rivers, lakes, or streams.[33]

during that visit. This will allow patients to make decisions regarding their own health and allows them to seek treatment after the team's visit. This should be discussed with local surgeons assuming care of the patient postoperatively.[11] Available treatment options and risks should be thoroughly reviewed with patients; they should also be informed about with whom they can follow up. Informed consent sheets should be provided and signed by the patients. Copies of the signed informed consent forms should be kept by the team and by the local practitioner who will follow the patients.

Providing treatment that follows the standard of care should always be the top priority. In addition to operating within boundaries and prudent case selection, this also includes exercising cultural competence, use of nonexpired, noncontaminated supplies, and use of sterile technique.[38] Failure to address these factors may lead to patient harm, violating the principle of nonmaleficence. Although operating conditions may be not equal

to those in high-income countries, it does not mean that the quality of care should be subpar. Team members should never speak negatively of the local accommodations. They should also never vocalize comparisons between facilities at home and those provided by the local hosts. As noted earlier, social media posts by team members should be first vetted by team leadership and should comply with HIPAA (Health Insurance Portability and Accountability Act) and Protected Health Information standards for patient privacy. Graphic surgical photos should never be posted.

DETERMINING THE MISSION'S SUCCESS

Although it is not uncommon to see reports from mission groups on numbers of patients treated or the dollar amount of supplies provided to these patients, neither of these values gives information regarding short- or long-term results, nor the true impact of the mission on the local community. The success of a mission should be determined by the quality of care provided and the impact it has on the community, not by the quantity of patients treated. When evaluating the mission's success, it is important to have a specific working definition; this can vary from location to location and should be based on the needs of that community. The definition of success should include measures of cost-efficiency, access to care issues, and progress made toward long-term solutions for the region.[11] This brings attention to 2 key points: (1) the increased need for research in the area of global surgery, and (2) the need to work closely with the locals for the purpose of achieving sustainability.

Data collection throughout the mission trip is critical for the development of the mission and can help determine the mission's outcomes.[19,39] Although available literature on global surgery is increasing, research addressing the need for and success of international surgical mission trips is lacking.[39] Research to date has focused on measurements of disease burden, models of surgical care implementation, development of cost-effective equipment, evaluation of team readiness before deployment, and other areas.[19] Ultimately this information can be used for a myriad of purposes, including accurate determination of mission outcomes, assessment of local needs, improvements in care and cost-efficiency, and long-term sustainability.

Whereas short-term missions provide necessary services at a given time, long-term sustainable missions maintain the benefits provided and can improve the region's medical self-sufficiency.[19] Delivery of care through a short-term mission may not always be beneficial to the receiving population; they do not address underlying socioeconomic problems, such as poverty or government corruption.[11] Additionally, if the surgical care provided cannot be followed up or is only available sporadically, it is possible that the presence of the mission can ultimately reduce the quality of medical care in that region. The key to long-term success is the establishment of the mission in conjunction with the local practitioners and community. This may include the incorporation of training programs for local practitioners,

Table 2
Sample timeline for planning a mission trip to Kingston, Jamaica

Timeline	Tasks
October/November/December 2016	Identify population or mission group that practitioner seeks to assist Identify needed surgical supplies and equipment. Create a master list to share with supporting leaders Meet local contacts to determine their needs and requests for the trip. Go over the master list with them to make appropriate adjustments If possible, visit work sites and commence establishing the clinic design and workflow if one does not already exist. Determine the number of needed team members and what volunteers are available from the local population Begin contacting companies/dentists for needed instruments and supplies. Determine funds needed to purchase the supplies and instruments and begin fundraising Begin recruiting team members
January/February/March/April 2017	Continue contacting companies/dentists for needed instruments and supplies. Begin/continue fundraising activities. Collect supplies from companies and keep a list of all supplies and funds acquired Finalize team, and create roster and WhatsApp group (or preferred method of communication). Submit all requested documentation to government officials or local contacts as soon as possible Host monthly meetings or post memos to educate and train team members as soon as final roster is established. Information regarding flights, vaccinations, travel advisories, emergency management, and designated responsibilities should be disseminated Develop system for cataloging borrowed instruments Identify volunteers/spaces for supply storage Determine how supplies will be shipped to target destination.
May/June 2017	Finalize budget from acquired funds. Contact companies to purchase supplies that are still needed. If sufficient funds are raised, purchase supplies by late June Confirm that team members have secured travel health and emergency evacuation insurance Confirm malpractice insurance requirement and coverage
Early July 2017	Latest time to order needed supplies. Deliver ordered supplies to storage site on arrival Have master list with all supplies ready for delivery to customs
August 2017 Before leaving for Jamaica	Lead the established team in packing suitcases Keep master list of which supplies are carried in which suitcases
August 2017 Returning from Jamaica	Make sure instruments are returned to lenders Debrief with team regarding mission success. Identify areas of needed improvement and successfully implemented strategies Catalog and store remaining supplies for future trips

Courtesy of Victoria A. Mañón, DDS, Houston, TX.

providing maintainable equipment or supplies to local clinics, or adding local surgeons to the mission's team.[19] Investment of local resources allows the community to improve at their socioeconomic level, in comparison with providing equipment or services that are only maintainable while the foreign team is present. Rather than create dependence, the ultimate goal should be to create a program whereby the local community is able to better care for itself once the mission team leaves.

SUMMARY

The planning and execution of an international surgical mission trip involves the consideration of various clinical and nonclinical factors, meticulous planning, and determination. Planning takes months and all steps need to be carefully outlined in the form of a timeline document. An example of such a timeline for an oral surgical mission trip to Jamaica is provided in **Table 2**.

DISCLOSURE

The authors have nothing to disclose.

REFERENCES

1. World Health Organization. Oral health. Available at: https://www.who.int/news-room/fact-sheets/detail/oral-health. Accessed December 14, 2019.

2. Warnakulasuriya S. Causes of oral cancer—an appraisal of controversies. Br Dent J 2009;207(10): 471–5.

3. Mehanna H, Beech T, Nicholson T, et al. Prevalence of human papillomavirus in oropharyngeal and non-oropharyngeal head and neck cancer—systematic review and meta-analysis of trends by time and region. Head Neck 2013;35(5):747–55.

4. Petti S, Glendor U, Andersson L. World traumatic dental injury prevalence and incidence, a meta-analysis. One billion living people have had traumatic dental injuries. Dent Traumatol 2018;34(2): 71–86.

5. Modell B. Epidemiology of oral clefts 2012: an international perspective. In: Cobourne MT, editor. Cleft lip and palate. Epidemiology, aetiology and treatment.Frontiers in oral biology, vol 16. Basel (Switzerland): Karger; 2012. p. 1–18.

6. World Health Organization. Density of dentistry personnel (total number per 1000 population, latest available year). 2018. Available at: https://www.who.int/gho/health_workforce/dentistry_density/en/. Accessed December 16, 2019.

7. Ferlay J, Colombet M, Soerjomataram I, et al. Estimating the global cancer incidence and mortality in 2018: GLOBOCAN sources and methods. Int. J. Cancer 2019;144:1941–53.

8. GBD 2016 Disease and Injury Incidence and Prevalence Collaborators. Global, regional, and national incidence, prevalence, and years lived with disability for 328 diseases and injuries for 195 countries, 1990-2016: a systematic analysis for the Global Burden of Disease Study 2016. Lancet 2017;390(10100):1211–59.

9. Hosseinpoor AR, Itani L, Petersen PE. Socio-economic inequality in oral healthcare coverage: results from the World Health Survey. J Dent Res 2012; 91(3):275–81.

10. World Health Organization. Oral health services. 2016. Available at: https://www.who.int/oral_health/action/services/en/. Accessed December 14, 2019.

11. Suchdev P, Ahrens K, Click E, et al. A model for sustainable short-term international medical trips. Ambul Pediatr 2007;7(4):317–20.

12. Bauer I. More Harm than Good? The Questionable Ethics of Medical Volunteering and International Student Placements. Trop Dis Travel Med Vaccines 2017;3(1). https://doi.org/10.1186/s40794-017-0048-y.

13. Caldron PH, Impens A, Pavlova M, et al. A systematic review of social, economic and diplomatic aspects of short-term medical missions. BMC Health Serv Res 2015;15(1). https://doi.org/10.1186/s12913-015-0980-3.

14. Barnett T, Tumushabe J, Bantebya G, et al. The social and economic impact of HIV/AIDS on farming systems and livelihoods in rural Africa: some experience and lessons from Uganda, Tanzania, and Zambia. J Int Dev 1995;7(1):163–76.

15. Niyonkuru F. Failure of foreign aid in developing countries: a quest for alternatives. Bus Econ J 2016;7(3). https://doi.org/10.4172/2151-6219.1000231.

16. Watson DA, Cooling N, Woolley IJ, et al. Healthy, safe and effective international medical student electives: a systematic review and recommendations for program coordinators. Trop Dis Travel Med Vaccines 2019;5(1). https://doi.org/10.1186/s40794-019-0081-0.

17. Johnston N, Sandys N, Geoghegan R, et al. Protecting the health of medical students on international electives in low-resource settings. J Travel Med 2017;25(1). https://doi.org/10.1093/jtm/tax092.

18. Imperato PJ, Bruno DM, Sweeney M. Ensuring the health, safety and preparedness of U.S. medical students participating in global health electives overseas. J Community Health 2016;41(2): 442–50.

19. Swaroop M, Krishnaswami S. Academic global surgery. Cham (Switzerland): Springer; 2016.

20. International Volunteer Trip Calendar. Available at: https://www.adafoundation.org/en/adaf-international-programs/international-volunteer-opportunities-se

arch/international-volunteer-trip-calendar. Accessed December 16, 2019.

21. Sykes KJ. Short-term medical service trips: a systematic review of the evidence. Am J Public Health 2014;104(7):e38–48. American Public Health Association. Available at: https://www.ncbi.nlm.nih.gov/pmc/articles/PMC4056244/.

22. Chapin E, Doocy S. International short-term medical service trips: guidelines from the literature and perspectives from the field. World Health Popul 2010; 12:43–53.

23. Members of the Christian Dental Society. Dental mission manual: for portable, short-term dental trips. Sumner (IA): Christian Dental Society; 2015.

24. Hupp JR, Ellis E, Tucker MR. Instrumentation for basic oral surgery, . Contemporary oral and maxillofacial surgery. 6th edition. St. Louis (MO): Elsevier; 2013.

25. Hupp JR, Ellis E, Tucker MR. Prevention and management of medical emergencies, . Contemporary oral and maxillofacial surgery. 6th edition. St. Louis (MO): Elsevier; 2013.

26. Schwei K, Cooper R, Mahnke A, et al. Exploring dental providers' workflow in an electronic dental record environment. Appl Clin Inform 2016;07(02):516–33.

27. Centers for Disease Control and Prevention. Travelers' health. Available at: https://wwwnc.cdc.gov/travel/. Accessed December 3, 2019.

28. US Department of State Bureau of Consular Affairs. Travel advisories. Available at: https://travel.state.gov/content/travel/en/traveladvisories/traveladvisories.html/. Accessed December 3, 2019.

29. Blazek J. IRS form 990: tax preparation guide for nonprofits. Revised edition. Hoboken (NJ): John Wiley & Sons, Inc; 2004.

30. Drucker PF, Hesselbein F. The five most important questions you will ever ask your organization. Hoboken (NJ): Wiley; 2015.

31. Kimmel PD, Weygandt JJ, Kieso DE. Reporting and analyzing inventory, . Financial accounting: tools for business decision making. 9th edition. Hoboken (NJ): John Wiley & Sons, Inc; 2019.

32. Hupp JR, Ellis E, Tucker MR. Infection control in surgical practice, . Contemporary oral and maxillofacial surgery. 6th edition. St. Louis (MO): Elsevier; 2013.

33. Centers for Disease Control and Prevention. Chemical disinfectants. 2016. Available at: https://www.cdc.gov/infectioncontrol/guidelines/disinfection/disinfection-methods/chemical.html#Glutaraldehyde. Accessed December 16, 2019.

34. Centers for Disease Control and Prevention. Sterilization. 2016. Available at: https://www.cdc.gov/infectioncontrol/guidelines/disinfection/sterilization/index.html. Accessed December 16, 2019.

35. Centers for Disease Control and Prevention. Peracetic acid sterilization. 2016. Available at: https://www.cdc.gov/infectioncontrol/guidelines/disinfection/sterilization/peracetic-acid.html. Accessed December 16, 2019.

36. UC San Diego. Autoclave overview. Available at: https://blink.ucsd.edu/safety/research-lab/biosafety/autoclave/. Accessed December 3, 2019.

37. American Dental Association. ADA Principles of ethics and code of professional conduct. Available at: https://www.ada.org/en/about-the-ada/principles-of-ethics-code-of-professional-conduct. Accessed December 18, 2019.

38. Alper J. Integrating health literacy, cultural competence, and language access services: workshop summary. Washington, DC: The National Academies Press; 2016.

39. Saluja S, Nwomeh B, Finlayson SR, et al. Guide to research in academic global surgery: A statement of the Society of University Surgeons Global Academic Surgery Committee. Surgery 2018;163(2):463–6.

Developing a Sustainable Program for Volunteer Surgical Care in Low-Income and Middle-Income Countries

Vennila Padmanaban, MD[a],*, David Hoffman, DDS[b], Shahid R. Aziz, DMD, MD, FRCS(Ed)[c,d,e,f], Ziad C. Sifri, MD[a]

KEYWORDS

- Global surgery • Outcomes • Oral and maxillofacial surgery • Humanitarian missions

KEY POINTS

- Volunteer medical missions to low-income and middle-income countries are an increasingly popular method of providing care to underserved regions of the world to address the substantial burden of untreated surgical disease.
- This text offers practical suggestions and tips in the preparation and execution of humanitarian surgical trips, based primarily on the experiences of 3 small-scale organizations with decades of experience.
- Important considerations include clinical concerns, optimizing patient safety, and host and volunteer logistical challenges.

Volunteer medical missions to low-income and middle-income countries have been a popular but unregulated method of providing care to underserved regions of the world as they work to improve surgical capacity. The recommendations put forth are a synthesis of best practices of 3 volunteer-based humanitarian organizations thought to be critical to the success of short-term humanitarian surgical trips. These surgical trips, often referred to as missions, are unified by the central aim of providing safe surgical care to underserved populations by small groups of medical professionals who volunteer time, skills, and resources. These efforts rely on mutual respect between the host and volunteer teams, based on communication and trust developed over a long time. Most importantly, to avoid unintended consequences despite good intentions, patient safety and cultural sensitivity are paramount.

THREE VOLUNTEER HUMANITARIAN ORGANIZATIONS

For 30 years, Healing the Children has been conducting humanitarian surgeries in South America and Central America; over the past several years, with successive visits and established relationships within the same community, a

[a] Department of Surgery, Rutgers New Jersey Medical School, 150 Bergen Street M232, Newark, NJ 07101, USA; [b] Department of Oral and Maxillofacial Surgery, Staten Island Oral Surgery, 56-C Mason Ave 3rd floor, Staten Island, NY 10305, USA; [c] Department of Oral and Maxillofacial Surgery, Rutgers School of Dental Medicine, 110 Bergen Street, Room B854, Newark, NJ 07103, USA; [d] Department of Surgery, Division of Plastic and Reconstructive Surgery, Rutgers – New Jersey Medical School, Newark, NJ, USA; [e] Update Dental College, Aichi Nagar, Khayertek, Turag, 1711, Dhaka, Bangladesh; [f] Smile Bangladesh, P.O. Box 1403, Mountainside, NJ 07092, USA

* Corresponding author. Department of Surgery, Rutgers New Jersey Medical School, 150 Bergen Street M232, Newark, NJ 07101.
E-mail address: vp379@njms.rutgers.edu

Oral Maxillofacial Surg Clin N Am 32 (2020) 471–480
https://doi.org/10.1016/j.coms.2020.04.003
1042-3699/20/© 2020 Elsevier Inc. All rights reserved.

comprehensive program has been established in Neiva, Colombia. The surgical team has evolved to a multidisciplinary team of pediatric orthopedic surgeons, oral and maxillofacial (OMS) surgeons, plastic surgeons, otolaryngology surgeons, anesthesiologists and certified registered nurse anesthetists (CRNAs), registered nurses (RNs), pediatricians, and other health care personnel. The surgeries are based in Neiva, a midsize city in the state of Huila, Colombia, populated by 1 million people. Areas of clinical focus include treatment of pediatric hip dysplasias, clubbed feet, cleft lip and cleft palate disorders, microtia, congenital and traumatic hand injuries, and a variety of other facial deformities. The medical team consists of local personnel from Neiva and other cities in Colombia as well as visiting surgeons from high-income countries.

The organization runs an annual bilingual speech therapy program concurrent with a teaching program for other speech language pathologists to provide therapy for pediatric patients with cleft-related conditions. As part of a multimodal approach to treatment, the organization has introduced cooking lessons for preparation of postoperative liquid diets for cleft-related surgeries. Families were provided with a blender, recipes, and produce; a well-known Colombian chef and his staff provided the lessons. Concurrently, the organization hosts a comprehensive preventative and therapeutic program for clubbed feet and hip dysplasia.

Smile Bangladesh (SB) is a New Jersey–based medical nonprofit, established in 2006. The organization's mission is to provide free-of-charge surgical care for indigent children and adults born with facial anomalies, specifically cleft lip and cleft palate and dentofacial deformities. One of the authors (SRA), a Bangladeshi American, founded SB after learning of the significant need for facial cleft surgery in Bangladesh—up to 300,000 children requiring surgery in the country. In 2005, Christina Rozario, at the time the Deputy Director of Impact Foundation Bangladesh, was contacted and a small cleft mission was planned to Kishoreganj, in rural northern Bangladesh, on Impact's floating hospital ship, the *Jibon Tari* (*Boat of Life*). The team consisted of 2 surgeons, 3 anesthesiologists, 4 nurses, and 2 surgical residents. Over the course of 3 surgical days, 40 primary cleft lips were repaired. This was a testament to the need for cleft surgery in rural Bangladesh and also supported the belief that most patients with cleft deformities often were unable to afford or access care. The organization evolved over the next 14 years, establishing 501(c)(3) status. In March 2020, SB completed its twenty-fifth mission and has provided 1600 free surgeries in Bangladesh, with cleft camps occurring twice per year and traveling to all corners of the country.

The International Surgical Health Initiative (ISHI) was founded in 2009 after the recognition of a need for elective general surgeries in austere settings outside of circumstances of acute crisis and disaster management. The organization is a 501(c)(3) nonprofit charitable organization, federally registered in Canada and the United States. Since its inception and maiden service trip to Guatemala in 2009, the nongovernmental organization (NGO) has hosted 30 short-term surgical missions to settings in Southeast Asia, West Africa, and the Caribbean. ISHI is focused primarily on delivering general surgical care inclusive of lifestyle-debilitating hernias; surgical oncologic care, such as soft tissue mass resections; gynecologic care inclusive of hysterectomies for uterine fibroids; and urologic care, such as hydrocele management and simple prostatectomies for benign prostatic hypertrophy.

Because the 3 organizations, described previously, render a diverse portfolio of surgical treatments in austere settings, the recommendations reflect the general needs of volunteer organizations applicable to various types of surgeries offered. The following topics are outlined as a general guideline:

1. Mission statement
2. Site location
3. Funding source and supply allocation
4. Team development
5. Case scheduling and comprehensive care provision
6. Safety, preparation, and emergency team planning
7. Medical records and documentation
8. Postoperative care and follow-up
9. Availability of patients and competing groups
10. Cultural norms and situational awareness

Mission Statement

Once a general concept is developed, it is imperative to develop a guiding statement that pertains to the effort and can be used to recruit qualified volunteers and engage donor agencies and stakeholders. The mission statement is intended to summarize clinical goals and convey information concerning programmatic intent, such as location and relevant patient demographics. To compose a mission statement that is aligned to host needs, it is beneficial to conduct surveys or interviews with local staff, via video conferencing or mobile connection. Based on the needs identified, the surgeries offered should be developed within the restrictions of the local environment. After clinical needs are established, the proposed roles of the team of volunteer should be defined and communicated clearly. The best intentions of a team prepared to provide a particular service may not be feasible or compatible with the local environment or may present undue competition with an ongoing program. Concurrently, guidelines should be established toward teaching local physicians based on their need and interest; this transfer of knowledge and skills improves the longevity of the impact of the trip.

Site Location

Site selection for the surgical trip should focus on 2 broad areas: (1) the community and its needs and (2) the volunteers and their needs with respect to safety and basic logistical considerations.

The community and its needs

An interested team must select a site location, a local hospital, or medical center with infrastructure to conduct surgery and obtain the support of the community at large. A relationship with the medical director of the hospital and the medical liaison for the community (potentially, local political leaders or informal community leaders) is critical to ensure that the team is welcome and that the community are willing and able to facilitate participation. A premission trip site evaluation can be helpful. This allows having a checklist of functional equipment needed for the trip.

As part of an initial needs assessment, confirm that a minimum, predetermined number of patients with the relevant clinical need are available (for example, a minimum of 50 surgeries) and that additional patients are invited for triage, because, unfortunately, some may be ineligible for safe treatment. The minimum number of cases is important to maximize the impact of the humanitarian trip and justify direct and indirect costs. With advanced planning, the visiting team may ensure that adequate supplies and infrastructure are available in the local community, for example, ensuring transfusion capability, if necessary. Conducting a clinical assessment about types of surgeries needed allows for adequate case selection, agreement with respect to types of surgery offered, and preparation of adequate supplies and personnel.

In addition, the authors advise coordination of plans preemptively with the local hospital administration. Requesting the presence of a local physician willing to complete an initial screen prior to the triage process helps optimize patient selection. Prior to trip preparation, it is important to ensure that the services rendered are welcome by pertinent local health departments or ministries. This includes arrangements with the government health organizations and provision of temporary licensure for practice. A formal memorandum of understanding between host and volunteer leaders that reflects goals, rules, and regulations is advised.

An additional consideration is that families may travel long distances and require accommodations and logistical support through the time frame of patient selection, convalescence, and postoperative care.

The volunteers and their needs

The volunteer team has basic needs with respect to safety and logistical considerations. In an effort to maximize volunteer safety, the authors recommend using the following questions to direct investigation of the host country and community:

1. Sociopolitical climate
   - Are there any Department of State travel advisories or restrictions?
   - Does the time of travel coincide with periods of potential political or economic unrest, such as elections or transitions of government?
   - Are there considerations with respect to visa and transit of health care providers as well as supplies?
   - Are there language considerations requiring translators?
2. Geographic and traveler's health considerations
   - Are the temperature and terrain navigable?
   - Is there a seasonally appropriate time to travel (eg, avoiding the rainy season or hottest temperatures of the year)?
   - What are the costs from the country of origin?
   - What is the distance from the host country's international airport or urban center to the hospital setting?
   - Are there special considerations with respect to vaccinations and disease prophylaxis?
3. Daily logistical needs
   - Is there a safe, convenient, and affordable facility for the team to be lodged?
   - Is there regular access to safe meals and clean water supply?
   - Is there convenient transport to and from the lodging to the facility?
   - What standards may assure personal safety (team escort or guard, curfew, and so forth)?

Funding Sources and Supply Allocation

Funding

Funds required for travel, lodging, local transportation, and medical supplies can be obtained via grants, fundraisers, or donations through individual and social media networks. Although patients are not charged routinely by the NGO, the hospital may need additional financial support for infrastructure use, diagnostic testing or inpatient stays, or provision of stipends for local staff. These needs require advanced consideration and planning.

Supply acquisition and transportation

In resource-constrained settings, patients or families are expected to purchase supplies required for surgery, inclusive of medications, sutures, and dressing supplies. To avoid straining the local ecosystem, organizations may establish systems of supply procurement and transport. Each volunteer may carry one check-in luggage item and is expected to check-in one 50-lb box of medical supplies on the aircraft. Requisite supplies are established and coordinated with each arm of the medical team (nursing, anesthesia, and surgery) and with the local team as to what is required and what may have to be purchased in-country. For example, narcotics are prohibited items of transport and have to be purchased locally. As part of supply planning, it may be beneficial to detail a packing list and, where applicable, obtain approval from local customs. A request of in-country supplies, such as bulk intravenous fluids, may be presented to the local team ahead of time, because some medications require purchase from regional hospitals and may not be available at the trip site.

Supplies are divided into durable medical equipment, such as patient vital sign monitors and electrosurgical units as well as surgical instruments, and perishable items, such as intravenous line placement items, syringes, and sutures. They are subdivided further into surgical supplies, such as instruments and sutures; anesthesia supplies, such as endotracheal tubes and spinal needles; and perioperative supplies required for patient care. The acquisition of supplies requires careful planning; however, they are available from donor organizations to hospital and private party donors. Supplies also may be available for purchase from medical device companies and third-party vendors. Electronic equipment should be compatible with host country voltage and available fuselage. Perishable supplies and medications should be unexpired to maintain efficacy, safety and sterility.

Team Development

Ideally, volunteers should have some experience traveling abroad and have clinical experience (that is, not recently out of residency/fellowship). Individuals should be professionally adaptable and ready and willing to perform in austere settings with limited resources. The number of volunteers on a surgical team is based on quantity of operating room tables that are available to the team; each table requires an anesthesiologist, surgeon, RN, and surgical assistant—either a resident or a cosurgeon. The hospital may support the team with local staff, precluding the need for a full complement of volunteers.

Additionally, health care personnel should be vetted for active licensing, skill level, and adaptability toward working in resource-limited settings. To foster team cohesiveness and expectations predeparture, a premission meeting and a team group communication thread, via email or text message, are advisable.

Team administrator/logistics

The team administrator or logistics component works to organize the team, supplies, predeparture, and in-country logistics. Ideally, individuals have language fluency in the host country. Additionally, the logistics team may help facilitate team dynamics by recognizing that the team may be composed of strangers and implementing cultural activities, educational programming, and team building. To foster flexibility and communication, teamwork in an austere setting may require flattening of the hierarchy that often traditionally is observed in the surgical community, and the involvement of nonmedical personnel can help facilitate this.

Nursing

Nurses provide a variety of essential services on surgical trips: they can be designated broadly as those in the operating room, such as circulators and scrub technicians, to postanesthesia care unit and recovery room nurses, to floor and ward nurses who also are responsible for preoperative care. Operations require varying skill sets and the nursing team must be appropriately coordinated; for example, post-prostatectomy patients requiring continuous bladder irrigation should receive the care of nurses comfortable with managing these systems.

Nurses are a critical element of discharge planning, care coordination, and patient counseling, particularly if a follow-up protocol is established. In many settings, nurses work closely with local nursing staff, particularly if overnight care is required with the assistance of local providers. They also may be extensively involved in teaching and training local staff.

Anesthesia

An anesthesia provider team can be a combination of an anesthesiologist, anesthesia technicians, and CRNAs. Certain countries may have limitations in scope of practice of allied health professionals and these should be understood in advance. Additionally, the use of anesthesia residents should be considered, with well-defined supervision.

In considering anesthesia, the team must consider that they may not be able to provide anesthetic care identical to that in high-income country modalities, resulting in limitations in parameters, such as CO_2 monitoring or high-technology capabilities. Additionally, medication and anesthetic availability may vary in the local context, and supplemental oxygen may be limited. The anesthesia and surgical teams must decide together what constraints are acceptable toward optimal patient safety. A pain regimen also should be established in coordination with the surgical team, because pain thresholds and narcotic sensitivities are variable among different populations.

The choice of modality of anesthesia may vary from what typically is rendered in high-income settings; for example, with limitations to monitoring capability, neuraxial regional anesthesia may be preferred. With limitations to postoperative pain administration after major surgery (for example, with the absence of epidural infusion), postsurgical peripheral nerve blocks can be an excellent supportive modality of postoperative pain control.

It is important that the visiting anesthesia team develop a good relationship with the hospital anesthesia staff and to involve them in the day-to-day operations of the mission. The local anesthesiologist is key to helping in difficult airways, emergencies, and overall care of patients. Additionally, the criteria for excluding a patient as a safe surgical candidate as well as the mechanism and possibility of canceling a patient's surgery always should be discussed. Finally, a rescue plan can be developed to address anesthetic or airway emergencies, including possibilities of a surgical airway and patient transfer contingencies, where available and applicable.

Surgical team

The surgical team should include a combination of skilled surgeons and residents or assistants. The key factor is to ensure surgeons are operating within their scope of practice. The cases of cleft lip and cleft palate treatment often become a philosophic debate in that a surgeon may not be doing much of this surgery at home but feels perfectly competent to provide this care in a volunteer overseas setting. This should be considered beforehand, and a team philosophy should navigate this problem easily and effectively. Although certain operations may not be a part of a surgeon's routine surgical practice, this should not necessarily limit their capacity to provide care, if they have had the prior training, necessary experience

and competence. There should be a designated surgical team leader to oversee scheduling and assignments.

Nonsurgical care

Certain teams may have roles for medical personnel overseeing evaluation of patients both preoperatively and postoperatively. Depending on the context, there may be additional roles for pediatricians, emergency physicians, internists, respiratory therapists, physical therapists, occupational therapists, and palliative care providers.

Case Scheduling and Comprehensive Care Provision

Case scheduling

To optimize case scheduling, anticipate potential process and systems challenges to occur on the first operative day and schedule accordingly. Additionally, the first operative day may be the first opportunity for the team to function cohesively, so it is prudent to avoid clinically vulnerable patients, such as the elderly and children, as well as complicated cases. Similarly, children and elderly are scheduled in the morning to avoid prolonged nothing by mouth (NBM) status.

To avoid overwhelming the postanesthesia care unit, minor and major cases of varying case duration are staggered. Also, it should be considered that cases may take longer in low-resource settings due to limitations, such as lack of electrocautery or limited instrumentation, staff, or supplies.

In certain circumstances, it is worthwhile to consider an add-on list of those patients with less urgent need who may be called electively to receive surgery in the event of an unexpected cancellation. The team may additionally provide consultation services in the emergency/outpatient department to offer diagnoses and referrals at the request of the host providers.

Comprehensive clinical care

Providing comprehensive care for a specific clinical pathology may present a challenge. These efforts may require returning to a hospital for several recurrent years to better incorporate some of the other services essential to comprehensive care. For example, in the circumstance of cleft lip and cleft palate, additional services, such as dentistry, orthodontics, speech pathology, genetics, and research, are essential and require time and resources to develop. There are many criticisms lodged that surgeons provide cleft lip and cleft palate repair and not address some of the other issues. Cleft care clearly includes speech therapy, hearing evaluations, and dentistry. When considering specialties, such as orthopedics or other types of facial reconstructive surgery, the same clearly holds true; postoperative therapy and rehabilitation have to be considered and their presence or absence must be accounted for.

Safety, Preparation, and Emergency Team Planning

Clinical preparation: rehearsals and dry runs

It is worthwhile to rehearse a sample operative day prior to beginning the operative week to ensure the new team understands patient flow and to identify potential gaps in knowledge, equipment, or processes. These sessions can be tabletop or a physical walk-through, with a volunteer impersonating a patient and team members reprising their roles. Often, these dry runs may illuminate overlooked components of the process, misunderstandings, redundancies, or inefficiencies that can be addressed prior to the first workday.

Similarly, at the conclusion of each workday, it is beneficial to conduct a debriefing session to allow the team to discuss errors or close saves and breakdowns in communication or process and to identify successes toward improving the next day and celebrating a successful workday.

Safety checklists

To decrease adverse events and errors and promote team cohesiveness toward safety in care of the patients, it is advisable to develop, communicate, and utilize simple checklists. The use of checklists standardizes critical elements that must occur before irreversible moments in patient care, such as skin incision and patient discharge. They are a convenient means of transferring key tasks from team to team and mission to mission and can be adapted to be appropriate to a particular clinical or geographic context. Sample preoperative and discharge checklists are shown in **Fig. 1**; they can be modified based on the mission specifics and printed on an index card.

Emergency planning

It is important to have a plan for emergencies established both prior to the visit and once the team has started providing services in a hospital setting. Things that should be considered: what to do if there is a medical emergency during a surgery; who the local doctors available to help out with a code or an emergent airway issue are; and availability and placement of an emergency cart. The team must consider what plans they have for an emergency should one occur during the operating schedule. It should not be taken for granted that there is something available. This should be thought of well in advance, and coordination and planning with the local hospital make taking care of an emergency more effective. These considerations are important

MRN_____	OR _____ Case _____
Pre-op Check List _____	**D/C Criteria** _____
Confirm:	Confirm:
o Identity/Index card	o Voiding
o Signed consent	o Pain controlled
o NPO	o Tol reg diet
o hCG? o No o Yes o N/A	o Ambulating
o Allergies?	o D/C instructions provided/ follow up appt discussed
o No o Yes _____	
o Tylenol 1g Time _____	
o Site marked _____	
o Checklist complete /OR Team notified	

Fig. 1. Sample preoperative and discharge patient checklists adhered to the back of a patient identifier index card.

particularly for postoperative care at nighttime; a volunteer member may be on call or required to stay at the hospital overnight to manage patients. Given the austerity of most of these sites, it is important to fully understand the limitations of the system. It may not be possible to scale-up patients to a higher level of care or to transfer patients to outside hospitals.

Medical Records and Documentation

It is important to have some type of medical record of a team's endeavors. These records are inclusive of case logs and mission reports and serve multiple purposes: the records are useful to the host medical system, to the volunteer organization, and to any donors or benefactors who require feedback.

To help identify patients, the ISHI has implemented a dual index card system. The cards issue identifiers for patients scheduled for surgery, including a medical record number, and record vital contact information as well as patients' procedure type and date of surgery. One index card is retained by the team, while the other, identically transcribed index card is given to the patient; the cards are matched on date of surgery to identify the correct patient. A sample patient index card is shown in **Fig. 2**.

The authors additionally implement a 10-page paper medical record system to track the progress of a patient during a hospital stay and to facilitate communication and record keeping. Every clinical area has a concise, 1-page documentation system capturing important information, that is, anesthesia vital sign and medication administration. The chart is inclusive of a history and physical form, a consent form, an operating room count sheet, an operative note, order sheets, and progress notes. As in traditional systems, the chart

accompanies the patient and allows providers to understand flow but is completed in a simple check system to maintain efficiency. A sample page is shown in **Fig. 3**.

In addition to organizational documents, host hospitals may have computer electronic medical records and want the team to provide records these patients. A designated resident or other provider may help streamline this process on a daily basis.

Postoperative Care and Follow-up

Depending on the scope of surgery and distance traveled to a hospital, patients may benefit from being monitored overnight to ensure they recover completely. The local nursing staff often is integrated into the system to care for patients overnight, which usually requires simple vital signs monitoring, pain management, and supportive care toward return to baseline function with respect to diet, urination, and ambulation. Physician and nurse team rounds then are conducted in the morning and afternoon. Discharge is conducted in coordination with local nurses to ensure questions and concerns are addressed appropriately.

If possible, a satellite team may be left behind with a provider to attend to immediate postoperative follow-up. This has been achieved for more than 5 years in West Africa and South America by the ISHI toward the attainment of short-term and long-term follow-up results. Where this is not practical or feasible, it is prudent to have local doctors included in the care of the patients who are willing to assume the postoperative care of the patients being treated.

Availability of Patients and Other Volunteer Groups

Visiting teams can have a problem with patient availability. In situations like cleft lip and cleft palate care, there often are many teams visiting a country and it is important to make sure that a team is not competing with a well-established program or a program that may be coming to that area a week of 2 before. It is frustrating for doctors to arrive at a site and they find out that 3 weeks prior, a big team had just come to the nearby city and had treated almost all the patients with the similar problems they are prepared to take care of. Checking the Internet for schedules of other medical volunteer groups who might be traveling or providing care to the proposed site can be helpful.

Cultural Norms and Situational Awareness

Through long-term relationships and contacts, the team can come to increasing awareness of the cultural norms that have an impact on delivery of

ISHI
INTERNATIONAL SURGICAL HEALTH INITIATIVE
ishiglobal.org

MRN: GH19 - 2

Patient Name: _____ Age/Sex: _____

Procedure: _____

Seen By: _____ Est. Duration: ____hr

Anesthesia: Local±Sed Regional Spinal General

Comments: _____

Surgery Date: Mon Tue Wed Thurs Fri

Surgery Time: Morning   Afternoon

Fig. 2. Sample patient identifier index card. (*Courtesy of* International Surgical Health Initiative, Jersey City, NJ.)

ISHI
ishiglobal.org

#SL19-_____

Progress Notes

Date/Time: _____

S: Pain – ☐ minimal/well-controlled ☐ moderate ☐ poorly controlled ☐ 0 - 10: _____
        ☐ Other: _____

Tolerating: ☐ Liquids ☐ Regular diet ☐ Not tolerating PO ☐ Not attempted PO
☐ Nausea ☐ Vomiting ☐ Flatus ☐ BM ☐ Ambulating ☐ Voiding

Other: _____

PE: General - ☐ AAOx3 ☐ NAD

Lungs - ☐ CTA ☐ Coarse ☐ Decreased: ☐ R ☐ L

Abd - ☐ Soft ☐ Distended ☐ Tender (location): _____ Other: _____

Wounds/Local - ☐ C/D/I ☐ serosanguinous staining ☐ saturated ☐ swelling ☐ induration ☐ pus

Other abnormal findings - _____

A/P: POD#____ s/p _____

☐ Advance Diet ☐ OOB/ambulate ☐ d/c foley

☐ Discharge to home

☐ Other: _____

_____

Signature/Date/Time: _____

Fig. 3. Sample patient progress note. (*Courtesy of* International Surgical Health Initiative, Jersey City, NJ.)

care in other settings. For example, in certain cultures, informed consent for surgery may involve engagement of the entire family in addition to the individual patient. In other contexts, patients may not know their precise age or prior medical history. In certain cultures, patients commonly chew kola nut, which has caffeine and other stimulant properties that contribute to baseline hypertension; elicitation of this information typically requires specific questions rather than asking broadly whether any herbal supplements are consumed. Agrarian patients undergoing hernia repair may find it financially prohibitive to abstain from heavy lifting for 6 weeks as advised in the postsurgical recovery period. Therefore, they may require additional education and counseling to prevent behaviors that may contribute to recurrence.

It is paramount to try to understand and observe local customs, for example, to avoid taking photographs without permission. Over time, with mutual exchange, trust, and continued collaborations, visiting teams may acquire a better understanding of these customs and their importance in the local society.

UNIQUE ASPECTS OF A FACIAL CLEFT SURGERY/MAXILLOFACIAL SURGERY MISSION

All of these points hold true in any global surgical mission. Unique to maxillofacial/facial cleft missions include the pediatric population treated as well as anesthetic and airway management concerns. The following points are based on 14 years of facial cleft surgery experience in rural Bangladesh:

1. Prior to visiting a new site—a site visit must be performed to assess primarily the anesthetic equipment, determine the number of tables that can be run simultaneously, and identify the closest blood bank. Most cleft lip/palate surgery is completed on infants and young children. Although the lip surgery is usually is benign and fast, with minimal blood loss, it is an infant undergoing anesthetic and it is the anesthesia that potentially causes significant morbidity or mortality. As such, the equipment must be evaluated and, if needed, updated equipment purchased. For palatal surgery, there rarely may be significant blood loss, which is especially critical in a child or infant, so identifying a blood bank is key.

2. Team selection—in accordance to global surgery tenets, surgical volunteerism is not medical tourism. As such, surgeons are selected based on facial cleft surgical experience. Anesthesia providers also are carefully selected, with pediatric anesthesiologists preferred. Furthermore, 1 to 2 more anesthesiologists than the number of operating tables should be brought, to ensure there is extra help if anesthetic issues are encountered in the operating room or recovery room. Recovery room nurses

also are carefully selected, with preference given to those with pediatric experience.

3. Patient selection—the first day of every mission is screening patients and setting up the operating rooms. Prior to the arrival of the surgical team, the host hospital preselects patients for screening and also obtains basic blood work. Selection is based on safety first—the surgeons review the blood work, health history, and also the patient's facial deformity to be sure that it can be corrected safely with the resources at hand. The rule of 10 is followed—hemoglobin level of 10 g/dl and 10lb (5 kg) of body weight, but impoverished Bangladeshi children may be malnourished—as such, it may take more than a year for a child to meet these criteria. Once a patient has cleared the surgeons, the anesthesiologists then evaluate the lungs/airway and review the chest radiograph. Once cleared by anesthesia, the patient then is scheduled for surgery.

4. Pre/intraoperative/postoperative planning—it is important to communicate to the host hospital and parents the NBM status of the child and also explain to the parents why NBM is so important preoperatively, so there is no secretive feeding of the patient. Typically, the first surgical day of the mission is on adult-sized children or older children so that the team can get accustomed to the facilities. The second day of surgery primarily is cleft palates, because these patients are left under observation for 2 days to 3 days postoperatively, checking for bleeding, airway compromise, and oral intake. Specific to cleft palates, the Dingman retractor is released hourly for 2 minutes to 3 minutes to allow lymphatic drainage of the tongue—this minimizes the risk of glossal edema and airway obstruction. Rural hospitals may not have electrocautery; as such, bringing disposable cautery and other hemostatic agents is helpful. A unique consideration to Bangladesh and other countries in South Asia, is that patients typically have small body habitus. As such, the endotracheal tubes brought that are based on US-sized patients may be too long; adjustments must be made to avoid intubating 1 lung. After surgery, the team does assess each patient as they would in the United States, and discharge is planned only when a patient is stable. Working with the physicians in the host hospital is important in this regard.

5. Education—global surgery provides an opportunity for experienced surgeons from both high-income nations and low/middle-income nations to exchange ideas. Education is a 2-way street. SB missions often are in rural parts of the country; local surgeons at the host facility are encouraged to operate with the team and SB is training a handful of surgeons to operate autonomously on facial cleft patients. In fact, 1 former site now has developed to the point where they no longer need an SB team—local surgeons now are comfortable in providing cleft care. In Bangladesh, OMS surgeons primarily are ablative oncologic surgeons—they have taught SB surgeons neck dissections. Conversely, Bangladeshi surgeons have extremely limited experience in orthognathic surgery. As such, SB has developed an orthognathic educational curriculum in conjunction with the Bangladesh Association of Oral and Maxillofacial Surgeons, in which local OMS surgeons are trained in orthognathic surgery.

SUMMARY

For many people, getting involved in volunteer missions can be the most rewarding service that can be provided in their profession. This discussion is meant as a guideline for help partaking in volunteer work. When people are asked why they do this, there often is no specific answer other than it is "a calling." For volunteer surgeons that have spent a professional lifetime volunteering several times a year, these trips have unique meaning that can be understood only by the person partaking. Whatever reasons motivate partaking, they all are good as long as it is understood that everyone is part of a team and that the goal is to provide medical care for people in need of the services. A notable quotation that epitomizes volunteer work is as follows: "You make a living by what you get; you make a life by what you give."

DISCLOSURE

The authors have nothing to disclose.

FURTHER READINGS

Bermudez L, Carter V, Magee W Jr, et al. Surgical outcomes auditing systems in humanitarian organizations. World J Surg 2010;34(3):403–10.

Johnston PF, Kunac A, Gyakobo M, et al. Short-term surgical missions in resource-limited environments: Five years of early surgical outcomes. Am J Surg 2019;217(1):7–11.

Butler M, Drum E, Evans FM, et al. Guidelines and checklists for short-term missions in global pediatric surgery: Recommendations from the American Academy of Pediatric Delivery of Surgical Care Global Health Subcommittee,

American Pediatric Surgical Association Global Pediatric Surgery Committee, Society for Pediatric Anesthesia Committee on International Education and Service, and American Pediatric Surgical Nurses Association, Inc Global Health Special Interest Group. J Pediatr Surg 2018; 53:828–36.

Meara JG, Greenberg SL. The Lancet Commission on Global Surgery 2030: evidence and solutions for achieving health, welfare and economic development. Surgery 2015;157(5):834–5.

Hodges SC. Anaesthesia and global health initiatives for children in a low-resource environment. Curr Opin Anesthesiol 2016;29(3):367–71.

Padmanaban V, Johnston P, Gyakobo M, et al. Long-term follow-up of humanitarian surgeries: outcomes and patient satisfaction in rural Ghana. J Surg Res 2020;246:106–12.

Padmanaban V, Tran A, Johnston P, et al. Gender equity in humanitarian surgical outreach: a decade of volunteer surgeons. J Surg Res 2019;244:343–7.

Shrime MG, Sleemi A, Ravilla TD. Charitable platforms in global surgery: a systematic review of their effectiveness, cost-effectiveness, sustainability, and role training. World J Surg 2015;39(1):10–20.

Torchia MT, Schroder LK, Hill BW, et al. A patient follow-up program for short-term surgical mission trips to a developing country. J Bone Joint Surg Am 2016; 98(3):226–32.

The History and Mission of Smile Train, a Global Cleft Charity

Angela S. Volk, MD[a], Matthew J. Davis, BS[a], Priya Desai, MPH[b],
Larry H. Hollier Jr, MD[a],*

KEYWORDS

• Smile train • Cleft lip • Cleft palate • Global surgery • Global cleft surgery

KEY POINTS

- Smile Train, founded in 1999, is an international children's charity providing comprehensive cleft care to children around the world.
- Smile Train improves access to safe and affordable surgical care and anesthesia to help children with clefts receive treatment in the developing world.
- Smile Train uses a sustainable partnership model to strategically allocate resources maintaining a bi-directional exchange with local medical professionals.
- Smile Train has expanded its reach to more than 90 countries, partnering with more than 1100 hospitals and over 2100 medical professionals, to support more than 1.5 million cleft surgeries to date.

BACKGROUND

Cleft lip and/or palate (CLP) is a common congenital anomaly contributing significantly to the global burden of disease.[1] It is estimated that 1 child out of every 700 live births is affected with a CLP. Globally, more than 200,000 children are born with a cleft each year.[2–4] Although mortality rates from CLP are generally low in the developed world, these rates are higher in developing nations, and without timely surgical treatment children may suffer from feeding difficulties, impaired speech and language development, recurrent infections, and lifelong emotional and social distress.[5] Because of higher prevalence rates and disparities in access to safe, affordable, and timely surgical and anesthesia care, a disproportionately high number of children with unrepaired CLPs reside in low- and middle-income countries (LMICs).[2,6,7] Given the challenges associated with providing quality health care in LMICs, the estimated global backlog of unrepaired cleft disease ranges from 400,000 to

2 million cases worldwide.[2,3] This number remains alarmingly high because of the many barriers children in LMICs face to accessing care, including financial constraints, difficulty finding transportation to health care facilities, and the lack of surgical infrastructure and specialty-trained surgeons in their local communities.[1,2,8,9] To ameliorate the burden of cleft disease, Smile Train, an international children's charity, used a sustainable partnership model to provide comprehensive cleft care (CCC) to children in need around the world.

HISTORY AND PARTNERSHIP

Smile Train was founded in 1999 by a software entrepreneur, Charles B. Wang. Wang's singular focus for the organization was to ensure that any child across the world born with a CLP had the opportunity to lead a full and productive life. Before Smile Train's establishment most international cleft charities were operating under a model of mission-based care. This model involves the

[a] Division of Plastic Surgery, Department of Surgery, Texas Children's Hospital, Michael E. DeBakey Department of Surgery, Baylor College of Medicine, 6701 Fannin Street, Suite 610.00, Houston, TX 77030, USA; [b] Smile Train, 633 Third Avenue 9th Floor, New York, NY 10017, USA
* Corresponding author.
E-mail address: Lhhollie@texaschildrens.org

Oral Maxillofacial Surg Clin N Am 32 (2020) 481–488
https://doi.org/10.1016/j.coms.2020.04.010
1042-3699/20/© 2020 Elsevier Inc. All rights reserved.

deployment of surgical teams to LMICs to provide cleft repair surgeries for as many patients as possible during a brief timeframe. When the mission is complete and the surgical teams depart, patients unable to have their clefts repaired must wait for the next mission to receive treatment. Several studies have found that this model is unsustainable, because it is limited by high costs, the inability to provide long-term follow-up care, and the often unsafe surgical practices generated by a focus more on patient volume than on repair quality.[10–17]

Charles B. Wang envisioned a different model of international cleft care, one that would provide sustainable, affordable, comprehensive, and safe care to all children with CLPs. Instead of sending medical professionals to LMICs on time-constrained missions, Wang founded Smile Train based on the "teach a man to fish" proverb and developed a model of partnership with local medical professionals. The partnership model is based on bidirectional exchange; through education and training, these local providers are empowered to expand their capabilities to provide efficient, CCC to children in need (**Fig. 1**). Compared with the mission model, the partnership model has been found to be more sustainable, more cost-effective, provide higher quality long-term care, and augment the abilities of partner hospitals and the economies of partner countries.[12,18,19]

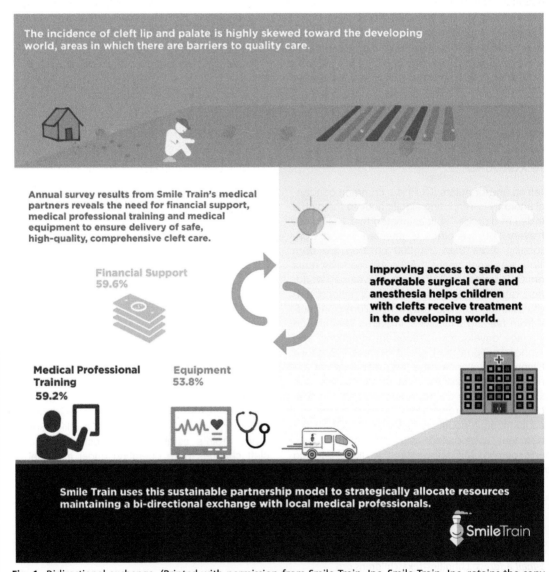

The incidence of cleft lip and palate is highly skewed toward the developing world, areas in which there are barriers to quality care.

Annual survey results from Smile Train's medical partners reveals the need for financial support, medical professional training and medical equipment to ensure delivery of safe, high-quality, comprehensive cleft care.

Financial Support
59.6%

Medical Professional Training
59.2%

Equipment
53.8%

Improving access to safe and affordable surgical care and anesthesia helps children with clefts receive treatment in the developing world.

Smile Train uses this sustainable partnership model to strategically allocate resources maintaining a bi-directional exchange with local medical professionals.

SmileTrain

Fig. 1. Bidirectional exchange. (Printed with permission from Smile Train, Inc. Smile Train, Inc. retains the copyright to this image.)

Smile Train aims to help local health care providers in areas with a high burden of untreated CLPs to be able to perform high-quality cleft repairs and offer CCC in a safe setting, without cost to patients. The ultimate goal is for local cleft care programs to become self-sustaining and able to address the needs of patients with CLPs around the world.

SAFETY

Central to its goal of providing safe cleft operations, Smile Train mandates that all partner hospitals adhere to a safety and quality protocol based on the World Health Organization and World Federation of Societies of Anesthesiologists international standards for safe surgery and anesthesia.[20] Each facility and surgical team are thoroughly audited and must maintain compliance with these protocols to receive continued support from Smile Train.[13] Systems have been developed to track the quality and impact of Smile Train's treatment mechanism, including partner surveys and programmatic review of quality assurance data.[21] This process ultimately improves more than just cleft care. By making the necessary changes to comply with the World Health Organization/World Federation of Societies of Anesthesiologists specifications, Smile Train partner hospitals in LMICs have seen a hospital-wide elevation in quality standards, protocols, and medical infrastructure.[19] Smile Train cleft programs have been active in 90 countries around the world, and the positive effects of partnering with Smile Train are widely visible to the local medical community and the local population. As a result, consistent partnership requests have led to steady growth in the number of active partner hospitals.[13]

COMPREHENSIVE CLEFT CARE

Cleft management does not end with the surgical repair; often a multidisciplinary approach with CCC is required by patients with CLP to achieve optimal outcomes and treatment goals throughout adulthood. CCC is defined as the provision of all necessary services to ensure successful CLP repair and total rehabilitation for patients. The main challenges toward offering CCC in developing countries include limited numbers of trained professionals in all different areas of CLP care, inadequate or outdated equipment and supplies, and patient difficulty returning for regular follow-up.

Because of its singular focus on cleft care and a partnership-based approach, Smile Train is able to address far more than just the surgical aspects of caring for patients with CLPs. In addition to surgeons and other medical professionals, Smile Train partners with CCC professionals, such as speech therapists, orthodontists, nutritionists, and psychosocial support providers.[13,18,19] Smile Train also funds important services for patients with CLP and their families that allows them to access CCC, including transportation, food, and housing costs.[13,18,19,22]

Education and Training

Empowering local medical professionals is crucial to Smile Train's partnership model. Smile Train approaches international cleft care by using and improving on existing local medical infrastructure and surgical training programs. After potential hospitals and surgical teams are identified, either by regional staff or by hospital self-volunteering, Smile Train helps to increase these teams' capacity and strengthens existing health care systems through parthership.[19]

For partner surgeons, Smile Train provides hands-on surgical training and education, exchanges with other partners, and conference and workshop support. Specific training courses also exist for speech pathologists, nutritionists, nurses, and anesthesia providers. To promote global conversations on cleft care, Smile Train provides scholarships for partner care providers to attend conferences and workshops. To date, Smile Train has supported greater than 1500 training programs and events and greater than 30,000 training and education opportunities. In 2019 alone, Smile Train awarded greater than 100 scholarships to sponsor partner surgeon attendance of international conferences and symposia.

One example of a training program offered by Smile Train is the Safe Nursing Care Saves Lives workshop. Although postoperative sentinel events occur at low rates after cleft operations, they are frequently respiratory in origin and more likely to occur when nurses are the primary care givers.[23] Recognizing that in resource-limited settings, nurses may lack the abilities and confidence to provide optimal care following cleft surgery, Smile Train developed this training program to teach nurses the necessary skills to anticipate, recognize, intervene in, and reduce postoperative complications. Knowing that empowerment and high morale are drivers for successful nurse-led interventions, another goal of this program is to improve the (self-) perception of nursing capability. Since 2011, Smile Train has trained more than 1500 nurses from 24 countries in postoperative nursing care through the Safe Nursing Care Saves Lives initiative. This course has the potential to not only improve the postoperative care patients receive, but also to increase nurses' confidence and normalize nurse-led intervention in countries with historic stigmatization of the nurse's role. Additionally, the program's Train-the-Trainer design has proven to be cost-effective, customizable, easily disseminated, and scaled in a fashion consistent with providing a successful training program in LMICs.

Oral Health

Children with clefts have a propensity for oral health challenges, and are often limited by their ability to access safe, affordable, and quality oral health care.[24] CLPs make children more prone to suffering from poor oral health, including dental caries, dental anomalies, and tooth malposition. These challenges are often compounded by these children's marginalization and lack of access to care, which are largely caused by a combination of stigma, out-of-pocket-expenses, and geographic barriers to access.[8] Without proper oral health, the prognosis for a successful long-term outcome for children with clefts is compromised.[24,25]

As part of its commitment to empowering local partners to provide CCC, Smile Train has worked to raise visibility, awareness, and support for oral health. One particularly successful campaign was born through a partnership with GlaxoSmithKline (GSK).[26] GSK has harnessed its oral health care salesforce and dental networks to raise awareness of the complications associated with being born with a CLP and the accompanying increased risk of compromised oral health.[26] In 2017, Smile Train and GSK launched a toll-free telephone number in India for families affected by clefts to call and receive information about CLPs, including resources on optimal oral health challenges and care.[27]

Another important development is a new partnership among Smile Train, GSK, and the World Dental Federation. Over the next 2 years, a World Dental Federation–led project team, funded by GSK, will research and consolidate ongoing guidelines for optimal oral health and dental care for infants, children, and adults with clefts.[28] This partnership will empower providers globally to ensure patients with clefts can achieve improved oral health via prevention and access to dental services.

TECHNOLOGY

Smile Train has used several innovative technologies to provide training, support, and education to partners and patients around the world. Some examples of Smile Train's successful leveraging of technology to maximize program efficiency include the development of a centralized World Wide Web–based database, an online virtual surgery simulator, novel three-dimensional (3D) facial analysis software, and several mobile applications. These innovations are helping to simplify and expedite the process of cleft repair training and outcome analysis across international cleft care.

Smile Train Express

Regular, rigorous assessment of surgical outcomes is facilitated by and conducted through Smile Train's online patient database, Smile Train Express. This database provides a platform for Smile Train partners to securely upload patient medical records, photographs, and videos for surgery and CCC treatments. For surgery records, preoperative and postoperative clinical photographs are evaluated through panel review by craniofacial plastic and reconstructive surgeons. This process allows analysis of individual partner surgeons' outcomes to ensure quality, and it informs Smile Train's Global Medical Advisory Board and Regional Medical Advisory Councils (RMAC) on the education and training needs of specific partner surgeons.

Virtual Surgery Simulator

In 2013 Smile Train released a virtual cleft surgical simulator to enhance training programs for surgeons and serve as a continuing medical educational resource for experienced surgeons. The simulator is an open-access, Internet-based, interactive program providing video, audio, expert tutorials, and testing features, in addition to the interactive exploration and simulation of surgical procedures.[29] Available in English, Mandarin, Spanish, Portuguese, and French, this simulator is currently being used in greater than 140 countries worldwide.

Three-Dimensional Facial Shape Analysis

In collaboration with researchers from the University of Glasgow and a startup company called NCTECH, Smile Train has developed a novel 3D facial analysis tool that is used to assess outcomes of cleft repair surgeries. A user-friendly, inexpensive digital 3D camera has been designed specifically for this project. Using this camera, researchers are able to make 3D statistical models of human faces using more than 1000 points, compared with the 23 points used by similar products when reviewing two-dimensional preoperative and postoperative photographs. These 3D facial shape analyses will provide surgeons with immediate and informative feedback on their cleft repair outcomes.

Mobile Device Development

In collaboration with a mobile tech company, Smile Train is working to develop an adapter that allows nasoendoscopes to be attached to mobile devices. The images captured by the endoscope can then be analyzed by a smartphone application to help guide treatment decisions. Together, these tools hold the potential for providers to visualize if/when speech therapy and/or corrective surgery for velopharyngeal insufficiency are necessary for patients with cleft palate, without the need for cumbersome and expensive endoscopy equipment. A pilot of these mobile nasoendoscopes is currently underway at a Smile Train partner facility in India.

Mobile Speech Application

Smile Train has also created mobile and Internet-based applications to assist in the provision of cleft speech services. Using the Speech Games & Practice English-language application and the Habla y Lenguaje Spanish-language application, children can participate in fun interactive stories, songs, and games to help improve speech. Additionally, an application has been designed for speech providers to help capture audio of patients to track the progress of speech services. These applications have been downloaded greater than 16,000 times across greater than 16 countries.

IMPACT

Smile Train is currently the world's largest cleft charity, dedicated to transforming the lives of patients with CLP around the world. By training local providers to perform cleft operations and to pass this knowledge along to their colleagues, Smile Train partners go on to train other medical providers, creating a long-term, sustainable system to consistently address CLPs on a global scale. Since its establishment, Smile Train has expanded its reach to more than 90 countries (**Fig. 2**), partnering with more than 1100 hospitals and more than 2100 medical professionals. More than 1.5 million Smile Train–supported cleft surgeries have been performed to date, which has significantly closed the gap between the annual number of new cleft patients born and the number of primary cleft repairs provided (**Fig. 3**).

Enormous economic benefits have resulted from providing cost-effective, comprehensive interventions to decrease the global burden of cleft disease. A 2016 study conducted by experts from Harvard Medical School's Program in Global Surgery and Social Change determined that the approximately $250 cost of a single cleft surgery translates to a 168-times return on investment when considering the destigmatization and overall health improvement experienced by Smile Train patients. Cumulatively, the global economic benefit of Smile Train's efforts to date has been estimated at up to $20 billion (**Fig. 4**).[30]

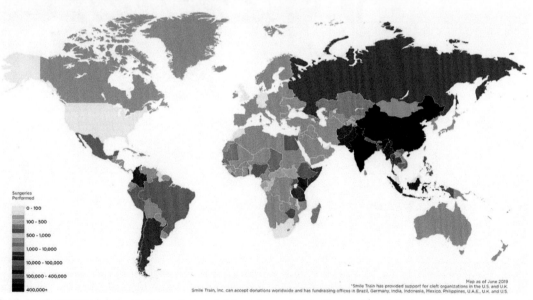

Surgeries Performed

0 - 100
100 - 500
500 - 1,000
1,000 - 10,000
10,000 - 100,000
100,000 - 400,000
400,000+

Smile Train, Inc. can accept donations worldwide and has fundraising offices in Brazil, Germany, India, Indonesia, Mexico, Philippines, U.A.E., U.K. and U.S.

*Smile Train has provided support for cleft organizations in the U.S. and U.K.

Map as of June 2019

Fig. 2. Smile Train's global presence, color-coded based on number of surgeries performed per country. (Printed with permission from Smile Train, Inc. Smile Train, Inc. retains the copyright to this image.)

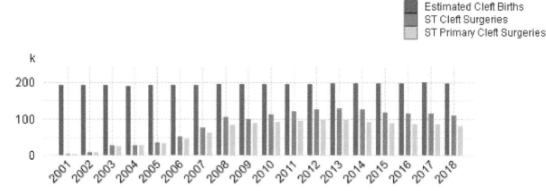

Fig. 3. Global coverage of new cleft cases by Smile Train partner surgeons, 2001 to 2018. ST, Smile Train. (Printed with permission from Smile Train, Inc. Smile Train, Inc. retains the copyright to this image.)

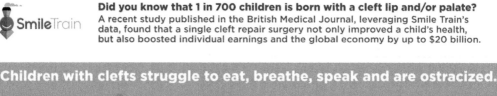

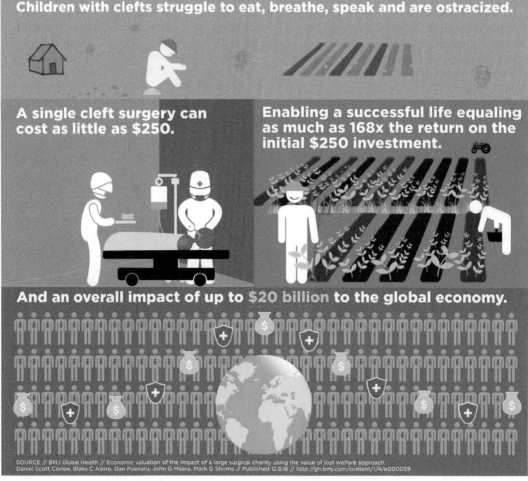

Fig. 4. The economic impact of Smile Train. (Printed with permission from Smile Train, Inc. Smile Train, Inc. retains the copyright to this image.)

FUTURE PARTNERSHIPS

Reflecting on the trajectory of Smile Train's impact on international cleft care, the scale of its success is attributable to partnering and collaborating with local surgeons and health care providers. Looking forward, Smile Train plans to take steps toward further solidifying these local partnerships. A United States–based Medical Advisory Board has historically advised Smile Train on its programs with input from RMACs, comprised of local surgeons, anesthesiologists, speech pathologists, orthodontists, psychosocial experts, nutritionists, and research experts, based in the countries with the largest Smile Train programs: China and India. However, Smile Train has come to realize that this model does not maximally take into account the unique nuances and challenges present in all of the regions where Smile Train has a presence. As such, in 2013 Smile Train began to expand the number of RMACs by creating additional councils in Brazil, Mexico, Africa, and most recently in Spanish-speaking South America. Each RMAC is tasked with helping Smile Train regional staff with program management and providing advice and guidance to Smile Train's Global Medical Advisory Board as it relates to investments in education and training, safety audits, and quality assurance of all cleft treatment services. In the spring of 2020, Smile Train will host a Global Cleft Summit that brings all of these regional advisors together to learn from one another and advance international cleft care through collaboration and discussion. These efforts exemplify Smile Train's deep understanding of the critical importance of partnership.

SUMMARY

Since 1999, Smile Train has maintained a singular focus on cleft care through partnership, enabling the organization to extend its efforts beyond the surgical repair of clefts to also support the provision of consistent, safe, and high-quality health care to patients around the world. By prioritizing safety, Smile Train has elevated the quality of care not only for patients with CLP, but also for every single patient seeking care at Smile Train partner hospitals. Moreover, for patients with CLPs, this care model has expanded beyond surgical care to include all aspects of CCC, from providing ancillary services and basic needs for families to bringing innovative technologies to the field. In terms of surgical and economic impact, Smile Train's efforts have been enormous, far-reaching, and most importantly, tangible on the smiling faces of more than 1 million children around the world.

DISCLOSURE

P. Desai is the Senior Director of Medical Programs at Smile Train—this is a paid position. Dr L.H. Hollier Jr is the Chairman of Smile Train's Medical Advisory Board—this is a volunteer position. The other authors have nothing to disclose.

REFERENCES

1. Bickler SN, Weiser TG, Kassebaum N, et al. Global burden of surgical conditions. In: Debas HT, Donkor P, Gawande A, et al, editors. Essential surgery: disease control priorities, vol. 1, 3rd edition. Washington, DC: The International Bank for Reconstruction and Development/The World Bank (c); 2015. p. 19–40.
2. Farmer D, Sitkin N, Lofberg K, et al. Surgical interventions for congenital anomalies. In: Debas HT, Donkor P, Gawande A, et al, editors. Essential surgery: disease control priorities, vol. 1, 3rd edition. Washington, DC: The International Bank for Reconstruction and Development/The World Bank (c); 2015. p. 129–50.
3. Poenaru D. Getting the job done: analysis of the impact and effectiveness of the SmileTrain program in alleviating the global burden of cleft disease. World J Surg 2013;37(7):1562–70.
4. Prevalence at birth of cleft lip with or without cleft palate: data from the International Perinatal Database of Typical Oral Clefts (IPDTOC). Cleft Palate Craniofac J 2011;48(1):66–81.
5. Jenny HE, Massenburg BB, Saluja S, et al. Efficacy of facilitated capacity building in providing cleft lip and palate care in low- and middle-income countries. J Craniofac Surg 2017;28(7):1737–41.
6. Higashi H, Barendregt JJ, Kassebaum NJ, et al. The burden of selected congenital anomalies amenable to surgery in low and middle-income regions: cleft lip and palate, congenital heart anomalies and neural tube defects. Arch Dis Child 2015;100(3):233–8.
7. Meara JG, Leather AJ, Hagander L, et al. Global Surgery 2030: evidence and solutions for achieving health, welfare, and economic development. Lancet 2015;386(9993):569–624.
8. Massenburg BB, Jenny HE, Saluja S, et al. Barriers to cleft lip and palate repair around the world. J Craniofac Surg 2016;27(7):1741–5.
9. Yao CA, Swanson J, Chanson D, et al. Barriers to reconstructive surgery in low- and middle-income countries: a cross-sectional study of 453 cleft lip and cleft palate patients in Vietnam. Plast Reconstr Surg 2016;138(5):887e–95e.
10. de Buys Roessingh AS, Dolci M, Zbinden-Trichet C, et al. Success and failure for children born with facial clefts in Africa: a 15-year follow-up. World J Surg 2012;36(8):1963–9.

11. DeCamp M. Scrutinizing global short-term medical outreach. Hastings Cent Rep 2007;37(6):21–3.

12. Kantar RS, Cammarata MJ, Rifkin WJ, et al. Foundation-based cleft care in developing countries. Plast Reconstr Surg 2019;143(4):1165–78.

13. Louis M, Dickey RM, Hollier LH Jr. Smile Train: making the grade in global cleft care. Craniomaxillofac Trauma Reconstr 2018;11(1):1–5.

14. Persing S, Patel A, Clune JE, et al. The repair of international clefts in the current surgical landscape. J Craniofac Surg 2015;26(4):1126–8.

15. Semb G. International confederation for cleft lip and palate and related craniofacial anomalies task force report: beyond Eurocleft. Cleft Palate Craniofac J 2014;51(6):e146–55.

16. Shrime MG, Sleemi A, Ravilla TD. Charitable platforms in global surgery: a systematic review of their effectiveness, cost-effectiveness, sustainability, and role training. World J Surg 2015;39(1):10–20.

17. Sykes KJ. Short-term medical service trips: a systematic review of the evidence. Am J Public Health 2014;104(7):e38–48.

18. Hubli EH, Noordhoff MS. Smile train: changing the world one smile at a time. Ann Plast Surg 2013;71(1):4–5.

19. Purnell CA, McGrath JL, Gosain AK. The role of Smile Train and the Partner Hospital Model in surgical safety, collaboration, and quality in the developing world. J Craniofac Surg 2015;26(4):1129–33.

20. Gelb AW, Morriss WW, Johnson W, et al. World Health Organization-World Federation of Societies of Anaesthesiologists (WHO-WFSA) International Standards for a Safe Practice of Anesthesia. Anesth Analg 2018;126(6):2047–55.

21. Braun TL, Louis MR, Dickey RM, et al. A sustainable and scalable approach to the provision of cleft care: a focus on safety and quality. Plast Reconstr Surg 2018;142(2):463–9.

22. Gupta K, Bansal P, Dev N, et al. Smile Train project: a blessing for population of lower socio-economic status. J Indian Med Assoc 2010;108(11):723–5.

23. Kulkarni KR, Patil MR, Shirke AM, et al. Perioperative respiratory complications in cleft lip and palate repairs: an audit of 1000 cases under 'Smile Train Project. Indian J Anaesth 2013;57(6):562–8.

24. Chopra A, Lakhanpal M, Rao NC, et al. Oral health in 4-6 years children with cleft lip/palate: a case control study. N Am J Med Sci 2014;6(6):266–9.

25. Lages EM, Marcos B, Pordeus IA. Oral health of individuals with cleft lip, cleft palate, or both. Cleft Palate Craniofac J 2004;41(1):59–63.

26. Healthcare GC. GSK consumer healthcare announces partnership with leading cleft lip and palate organization smile train to bring comprehensive care to children born with clefts. 2018. Available at: https://www.prnewswire.com/news-releases/gsk-consumer-healthcare-announces-partnership-with-leading-cleft-lip-and-palate-organization-smile-train-to-bring-comprehensive-care-to-children-born-with-clefts-300683658.html. Accessed November 1, 2019.

27. Smile Train India launches a toll-free cleft helpline on National Cleft Day. 2019. Available at: https://www.smiletrain.org/media/press/smile-train-india-launches-toll-free-cleft-helpline-on-national-cleft-day. Accessed November 1, 2019.

28. Oral Health in Cleft Patients Project. 2019. Available at: https://www.fdiworlddental.org/what-we-do/projects/oral-health-in-cleft-patients-project. Accessed November 1, 2019.

29. Volk AS, Eisemann BS, Dibbs RP, et al. The utility of an open-access surgical simulator to enhance surgeon training. J Craniofac Surg 2020;31(1):72–6.

30. Poenaru D, Lin D, Corlew S. Economic valuation of the global burden of cleft disease averted by a large cleft charity. World J Surg 2016;40(5):1053–9.

Creating the Successful Global Maxillofacial Surgeon: A 35-Year Perspective

James E. Bertz, DDS, MD[a,1], Ghali E. Ghali, DDS, MD, FRCSEd[b],
Thomas P. Williams, DDS, MD[c,*]

KEYWORDS

- Global surgical outreach program • Global oral and maxillofacial surgery • Cultural and social norms

KEY POINTS

- The success of any global outreach surgical program depends on many factors including the preparation of the surgeons involved in the program.
- Surgeons preparing for global outreach programs often focus on surgical procedures or techniques as the most important aspect of the preparation for the program.
- Although surgical techniques including modifications made to accommodate the resources available to the program are important, just as important to success of the outreach program is the surgeon's familiarity with the language, cultural, and social norms of the host country or region.
- This article provides valuable information on these issues from three oral and maxillofacial surgeons who have been engaged in global oral and maxillofacial surgery outreach programs for decades.

Sister Teresa stated you have not lived until you have done something for someone who can never repay you. This is a premise for those who embark on a global surgical outreach program. There are many reasons one decides to participate on a program of this type. Helping individuals who do not have an opportunity to receive treatment should be the primary objective of all those who enlist to serve on an overseas outreach program. There is also a feeling that if you do not participate, someone else may not either. The many rewards for participating include developing a sense for volunteerism, helping those less fortunate, learning new surgical procedures, traveling to different parts of the world, and developing lifelong friendships (**Table 1**).

Education is an important aspect for oral and maxillofacial surgeons embarking on a global outreach program. Before leaving for the program the surgeon should familiarize themselves with knowledge of the country and region to be visited in terms of its geography, language, and culture. In addition, the surgeon must prepare with an appropriate medical evaluation and immunizations, travel medical and safety evacuation coverage, and liability insurance. Much thought should be given to the acquisition and logistics of transporting appropriate supplies and instruments dependent on the type of procedures to be performed. A significant consideration for surgeons embarking on their first overseas trip is to learn about the types of surgical procedures

[a] Department of Oral and Maxillofacial Surgery, University of Texas at Houston, Houston, TX, USA; [b] Department of Oral and Maxillofacial Surgery, LSU Health Sciences Center, Louisiana State University Health System, Shreveport, LA 71130, USA; [c] 1870 Links Glen, Dubuque, IA 52003, USA
[1] Present address: 3501 North Scottsdale Road, Suite #110, Scottsdale, AZ 85251.
* Corresponding author.
E-mail address: illinioms@aol.com

Oral Maxillofacial Surg Clin N Am 32 (2020) 489–493
https://doi.org/10.1016/j.coms.2020.04.011

Table 1
Reasons to pursue global surgery during training
1. Surgical altruism/philanthropy
2. Surgical education
3. Experience new cultures
4. Connect with colleagues globally

that are planned to be safely performed as part of the program.

Preparation for the program occurs in several other areas (**Table 2**). To begin, the resident/fellow junior surgeon should research the area where the mission will occur. They must have a valid passport. If a visa is required, application should occur well in advance of the trip. The sponsoring organization assists the outreach team with obtaining visas if they are needed. Virtually all countries require temporary licensure granted by the host country's Ministry of Health; therefore, copies of current licenses, diplomas, and evidence of board certification may need to be provided up to 6 months before departure. Outreach programs can occur in a hot climate and knowledge of the region's climate and time of the year influence the type of clothing needed. Often the team are guests at events of the city they are visiting that require appropriate dress. In most cases this does not require more than business casual; senior surgeons and mission administrators can provide recommendations in this regard. For daily travel to and from the hospital, it is beneficial to bring a small carry bag to transport items, such as scrubs, magnifying glasses, and reference texts. It is beneficial to inquire about the type of food provided to the group during their stay. Allergies may affect diet and it is always beneficial to bring snacks of some sort. It is also advisable to make copies of the individual's credit cards and passport so in the event they are lost, credit cards can be canceled and the passport replaced by the local embassy or consulate. This can easily be accomplished by using one's cell phone.

Surgeons traveling to an overseas site must be aware and sensitive of the culture of the country they are visiting. This ensures that the visiting team avoids behavior that might be interpreted as disrespectful by the team's host.

Bringing a camera for taking clinical photographs is a necessity. Today's technology facilitates this goal with much smaller equipment than was needed in the past. The surgeon should be aware of cultural sensitivities and should obtain permission before taking photographs. Permission should also be obtained before taking photographs of cultural sites.

Taking photographs of sensitive areas should not be done. During one of the author's (TPW) initial trips to Colombia, he was taking photographs of the hospital. Immediately adjacent to the hospital was a government building that was headquarters for DAS, the Colombian Department of Administrative Security, similar to our FBI. Immediately after taking photographs, he was confronted by DAS officials creating an uncomfortable situation that rapidly escalated. Only with the help of one of the local hosts was he able to keep his camera and film. Despite that particular experience, one of the many rewards of traveling on a global surgical outreach program is to share your experiences and photographs with colleagues, family, and friends.

Learning about the area where you will be traveling from guide books or Web sites provides interesting facts making one a more knowledgeable visitor. In addition, maps are beneficial. Exchanging currency should be accomplished at a local bank, which often have a better exchange rate than what is offered in airports. It is advantageous to plan to carry some local currency for tipping, taxis, and other situations. Credit cards are accepted at most local hotels and restaurants.

Many global surgery outreach programs that oral and maxillofacial surgeons participate in are focused on treating patients with cleft lip and palate deformities. It is therefore important for the surgeon to prepare by reviewing the altered anatomy and techniques used to reconstruct these defects. There are many textbooks addressing cleft surgery and these are a great starting point for learning.[1–5] Also available are videos where cleft surgical procedures can be visualized.[6,7] It may be beneficial to ask a colleague to observe and/or assist during a cleft lip or palate repair.

We suggest that the new surgeon know one technique for repair of unilateral and bilateral cleft lip deformities. In the authors experience, this should be the Millard technique, which is the most common technique used in the English-speaking countries and many others. This procedure has the objective of repositioning the muscles in proper position to allow normal function. The rotation of the nonclefted side repositions the orbicularis oris muscle in a more horizontal relationship; release and advancement of the clefted side provides the best opportunity for normal muscle function. In addition, repair of the lower lateral nasal cartilage on the clefted side provides the best chance to reproduce the normal anatomy of the nonclefted side. The Millard bilateral cleft

Table 2
Preparing for surgical mission

1. Review country to be visited
   a. Vaccines/immunizations needed
   b. Malaria prophylaxis
   c. Review Centers for Disease Control and Prevention country guidelines (https://www.cdc.gov/travel/destinations/list)
   d. Cultural issues: religion, language, alcohol restrictions, gender interactions
2. Purchase travel/evacuation health insurance
   a. Commercial
   b. Institutional
3. Surgical supplies and instrumentation based on needs
   a. Surgical scrubs
   b. Instrumentation: based on surgeries planned
   c. Personal protective equipment: masks, gowns, head cover, hand sanitizer, bug spray, and so forth
   d. Head light
4. Visa requirements: refer to embassy/consulate in United States for guidelines
5. Passport
   a. Ensure valid for at least 6 months
   b. Keep a copy of passport photograph page with family/friend in United States
   c. Keep copy of passport photograph page with you and in your email
6. Register with Safe Traveler Enrollment Program (https://step.state.gov/)
7. Have US embassy/consulate address/telephone number stored
8. Purchase international telephone access through your existing mobile phone carrier or bring an unlocked old mobile phone and purchase in-country a SIM card for said phone
   a. Allows for mobile phone access in country and smart phone use in areas where Wi-Fi is not available
   b. In-country SIM card purchase is done usually in arrival airport and is cheaper than international plans on US mobile phones
   c. International electrical adapters and portable chargers to keep electronics charged
9. Find out if accommodations have laundry facilities to reduce volume of clothing needed to travel
10. Suggested medications for travel to remote regions
    a. 2–3 days extra prescription medications
    b. Tylenol, nonsteroidal anti-inflammatory drugs (Motrin, Aleve)
    c. Hand sanitizer
    d. Insect repellant
    e. Benadryl/EpiPen, especially if food allergies
    f. Common cold medications
    g. Dental needs: floss, toothbrush, toothpaste
    h. Antibiotics
       • Amoxicillin or levofloxacin: for generalized antibiotic needs
       • Cephalosporin: for dermatologic infection/cellulitis
       • Azithromycin (Z-pack): for sinusitis or respiratory infection
       • Ciprofloxacin: for gastroenteritis treatment
       • Malaria prophylaxis as needed

repair allows for repair of the muscle beneath the prolabium with the goal of restoring function.[8]

The corresponding author's first trip (TPW) was 35 years ago to Villavicencio, Colombia with Healing the Children. The program was led by Dr Larry Herman and the team anticipated treating patients with primary cleft lip and palate deformities. Having limited experience treating cleft deformities at that point of his career, the corresponding author spent a significant amount of time by reading, attending meetings, and watching videos describing anatomy and surgical techniques.

However, there is no substitute for actually observing and assisting in surgical procedures. Only after several trips and multiple surgeries does the surgeon feel comfortable managing these patients as the primary surgeon. Oral and maxillofacial surgeons are familiar with the anatomy and possess abilities that make the acquisition of the cleft repair skill sets straightforward. To become competent, however, requires years of experience.

An excellent opportunity for senior OMS residents to participate in well-run and educationally

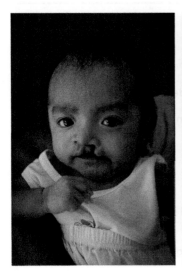
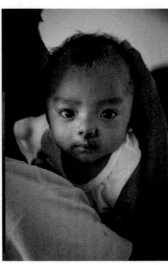

Fig. 1. Preoperative and one day postoperative views of unilateral cleft lip.

sound global surgery outreach programs is the Global Initiative for Volunteerism (GIVE program) initiated in 2018 and sponsored by the Oral and Maxillofacial Surgery Foundation. This program matches a senior oral and maxillofacial surgery (OMS) resident to a well-established surgical outreach program led by knowledgeable team leaders and also provides financial support for the resident to help cover travel and other expenses. Currently there are 10 approved mission programs that are available for residents to participate. These programs provide the opportunity for residents to learn the concept of volunteerism and have the opportunity to observe surgical procedures they may not have had the opportunity to assist in their training program. Types of problems treated on the 10 approved GIVE mission trips vary from reconstruction, treatment of pathology, ankylosis, and cleft lip and palate deformities.

A question often asked is should management of primary clefts be included as part of the core curriculum for OMS residency training. Currently not all the oral and maxillofacial surgeon programs offer the opportunity for a resident to participate in the treatment of craniofacial anomalies including clefts. Despite this there are several oral and maxillofacial surgeons who have the expertise and experience to teach residents in this discipline. Another consideration is for OMS residents to obtain credit for surgical experiences encountered during a global surgical outreach program, which is currently not in place. This will facilitate obtaining privileges and becoming an integral part of a cleft team.

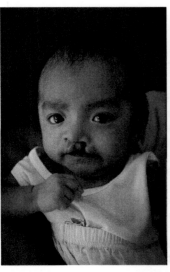
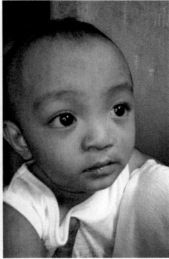

Fig. 2. Preoperative view and one year follow up. Surgery performed using the Millard Technique by author James E. Bertz.

When an individual participates in a global surgical outreach program, there are many rewards. The joy and satisfaction of helping individuals who do not have the ability to obtain surgical care is immensely gratifying. In addition, lifelong friendships are developed and provide the impetus to continue to participate. The friendships and satisfaction of shared experiences persist throughout one's lifetime (**Figs. 1** and **2**).

DISCLOSURE

The authors have nothing to disclose.

REFERENCES

1. Grabb WC, Rosenstein SW, Bzoch KR. Cleft lip and palate. 1st edition. Boston: Little, Brown; 1971.

2. McCarthy JG, May JW, Littler JW. 1st edition. Plastic surgery, vol. 4. Philadelphia: Saunders; 1970.

3. Bardach J, Salyer KE. Surgical techniques in cleft lip and palate. 2nd edition. St. Louis (MO): Mosby; 1991.

4. van de Ven B, Defrancq J, Defrancq E. Cleft lip surgery: a practical guide. Agave Clinic; 2008.

5. Bütow K, Zwahlen R. Cleft ultimate treatment: orofacial and cranio-maxillo-facial deformities. 2nd edition. Reach Publishers; 2016.

6. Cutting CB, LaRossa D, et al. Virtual surgery video, vols. 1, 2. New York City: Smile Train; 2007.

7. Rogers DJ, Hartnick CJ, Hamden US. Video atlas of cleft lip and palate surgery. San Diego (CA): Plural Publishing.

8. Millard DR. Cleft Craft: The Evolution of Its Surgery. Volume I-III. Boston: Little Brown; 1976, 1977, 1980.

Moving?

Make sure your subscription moves with you!

To notify us of your new address, find your **Clinics Account Number** (located on your mailing label above your name), and contact customer service at:

Email: journalscustomerservice-usa@elsevier.com

800-654-2452 (subscribers in the U.S. & Canada)
314-447-8871 (subscribers outside of the U.S. & Canada)

Fax number: 314-447-8029

Elsevier Health Sciences Division
Subscription Customer Service
3251 Riverport Lane
Maryland Heights, MO 63043

*To ensure uninterrupted delivery of your subscription, please notify us at least 4 weeks in advance of move.

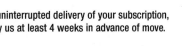

Printed and bound by CPI Group (UK) Ltd, Croydon, CR0 4YY

08/05/2025

01864691-0015

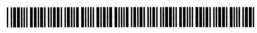